Drug Prescribing in Renal Failure

D1531008

For a catalogue of publications available from ACP-ASIM, contact:

Customer Service Center
American College of Physicians–American Society of Internal Medicine
190 N. Independence Mall West
Philadelphia, PA 19106-1572
215-351-2600
800-523-1546, ext. 2600

Visit our web site at www.acponline.org

Drug Prescribing in Renal Failure

Dosing Guidelines for Adults

Fourth Edition

George R. Aronoff, MD, FACP
Jeffrey S. Berns, MD, FACP
Michael E. Brier, PhD
Thomas A. Golper, MD
Gail Morrison, MD, FACP
Irwin Singer, MD, FACP
Suzanne K. Swan, MD, FACP
William M. Bennett, MD, FACP

American College of Physicians

Philadelphia, Pennsylvania

Acquistions Editor: **Mary K. Ruff**
Manager, Book Publishing: **David Myers**
Administrator, Book Publishing: **Diane McCabe**
Production Supervisor: **Allan S. Kleinberg**
Production Editor: **Scott Thomas Hurd**
Cover and Interior Design: **Patrick Whelan**

Copyright © 1999 by the American College of Physicians–American Society of Internal Medicine. All rights reserved. No part of this book may be reproduced in any form by any means (electronic, mechanical, xerographic, or other) or held in any information storage and retrieval systems without written permission from the publisher.

Fourth Edition

Printed in the United States of America
Composition by Fulcrum Data Services, Inc.
Printing/binding by Victor Graphics

American College of Physicians (ACP) became an imprint of the American College of Physicians–American Society of Internal Medicine in July 1998.

Library of Congress Cataloging-in-Publication Data

Drug prescribing in renal failure : dosing guidelines for adults /
    George R. Aronoff . . . [et al.]. — 4th ed.
        p.   cm.
    Includes bibliographical references and index.
    ISBN 0-943126-76-2
    1. Chronic renal failure—Complications. 2. Drugs—Prescibing—
Tables. 3. Drugs—Metabolism—Tables. I. Aronoff, George R.,
    1950-
        [DNLM: 1. Pharmaceutical Preparations—administration & dosage
tables. 2. Kidney Failure—drug therapy tables.   QV 16 D794 1998]
    RC918.R4D7   1999
    616.6'1061—dc21
    DNLM/DLC
    for Library of Congress
                                                    98-44099
                                                    CIP

The authors and publisher have exerted every effort to ensure that drug selection and dosage set forth in this manual are in accord with current recommendations and practice at the time of publication. In view of ongoing research, occasional changes in government regulations, and the constant flow of information relating to drug therapy and drug reactions, the reader is urged to check the package insert for each drug for any change in indications and dosage and for added warnings and precautions. This care is particularly important when the recommended agent is a new or infrequently used drug.

99 00 01 02 03 04/9 8 7 6 5 4

Authors

George R. Aronoff, MD, FACP
Professor of Medicine
Chief, Division of Nephrology
University of Louisville
Louisville, Kentucky

William M. Bennett, MD, FACP
Professor of Medicine and Pharmacology
Division of Nephrology and Hypertension
Oregon Health Sciences University
Portland, Oregon

Jeffrey S. Berns, MD, FACP
Clinical Associate Professor of Medicine
MCP Hahnemann University School of Medicine
Graduate Hospital
Philadelphia, Pennsylvania

Michael E. Brier, PhD
Associate Professor of Medicine
University of Louisville;
Department of Veterans Affairs
Louisville, Kentucky

Thomas A. Golper, MD
Professor of Medicine
Univeristy of Arkansas for Medical Sciences
Little Rock, Arkansas;
Chief Medical Officer
Renal Disease Management, Inc.
Youngstown, Ohio

Gail Morrison, MD, FACP
Vice Dean for Education
Director of Academic Programs
Professor of Medicine
University of Pennsylvania School of Medicine
Philadelphia, Pennsylvania

Irwin Singer, MD, FACP
Clinical Professor of Medicine
University of Miami School of Medicine;
Consultant
Miami Veterans Administration Medical Center
Miami, Florida

Suzanne K. Swan, MD, FACP
Associate Professor of Medicine
University of Minnesota Medical School
Division of Nephrology
Hennepin County Medical Center
Minneapolis, Minnesota

Preface

The fourth edition of *Drug Prescribing in Renal Failure: Dosing Guidelines for Adults* is an important text for physicians. Because the kidney eliminates many drugs, it is important for physicians to know how to alter the doses of medications in patients who have kidney disease. With the expansion of the available FDA-approved medications to literally hundreds and the aging of the U.S. population, the potential problems of under-dosing or overdosing medications in patients with kidney disease, including the treatment and cost implications, are proliferating. Over 40% of prescriptions are written for people over 65 years old, and kidney function is known to deteriorate with age. When an elderly patient is admitted to the hospital, there is a 30% likelihood that the admission is due to problems with the patient's medications. Furthermore, this revised edition emphasizes not only the need to recognize the medications that are eliminated by the kidney but also the importance of knowing the patient's glomerular filtration rate (GFR). Measurement of the level of serum creatinine alone is insufficient for a proper diagnosis, because a value of 1.4 mg/dL may indicate a GFR of 25 mL/min in a well-developed woman aged 75 years, whereas it may indicate a GFR of 125 mL/min in a well-developed man aged 25 years. This manual provides the physician with the knowledge to order the correct dose of medication for patients with kidney failure. This knowledge must be patient-specific and available at the point of patient care in the physician's office, the hospital ward, and the emergency department. Retrospective approaches to drug dosing in the pharmacy after the drug has been administered are inadequate.

Contents

Bibliography 99

Introduction

Uremia affects every organ system and every aspect of drug disposition by the body. The kidney is the major regulator of the internal fluid environment; therefore, the physiologic changes associated with renal disease can have pronounced effects on the pharmacology of many drugs. Clinicians must have a basic understanding of the biochemical and physiologic effects of drugs in patients with renal disease.

Bioavailability

The amount and appearance kinetics of a drug in the central circulation compared with those of a drug given intravenously define its bioavailability (1). Drugs given intravenously enter the central circulation directly and generally have rapid onset of action. Drugs introduced by other routes must first traverse a series of membranes and may need to pass through important organs of elimination before entering the systemic circulation. Only a fraction of the administered dose may reach the circulation and become available at the site of drug action.

Gastrointestinal absorption of drugs may be decreased in patients with uremia. Gastrointestinal symptoms are common in uremia, but there is little specific information about bowel function in patients with renal failure. The gastric alkalinizing effect caused by salivary urea that is converted to ammonia by urease or by the use of histamine H_2-receptor antagonists may decrease the absorption of drugs that are best absorbed in an acidic environment (2). This effect may be particularly important for patients receiving oral iron supplements, which require conversion by acid from ferrous to ferric forms for absorption. The ingestion of milk or other sources of multivalent cations (e.g., aluminum-containing antacids) may decrease drug absorption by chelation and by the formation of nonabsorbable complexes (3). In addition,

1

uremic patients have decreased small-bowel absorptive function (4).

First-pass hepatic metabolism may be altered in uremia. Decreased biotransformation may lead to increased amounts of active drug in the systemic circulation and enhanced bioavailability of some drugs. Conversely, impaired plasma protein binding allows more free drug available at the site of hepatic metabolism, increasing the amount of drug removed during the hepatic first pass. The interactions of absorption and first-pass hepatic metabolism are complex. It is not surprising that drug bioavailability varies more in patients with renal impairment than in patients with normal renal function.

Distribution

After administration, a drug disperses throughout the body at a given rate. At equilibrium, the apparent volume of distribution is the ratio of the amount of drug in the body to its plasma concentration. This ratio does not refer to a specific anatomic space but rather estimates the initial dose of a drug needed to reach a therapeutic plasma concentration. Highly protein-bound agents or those that are water soluble tend to be restricted to the extracellular fluid space and have small volumes of distribution. On the other hand, drugs that are highly lipid soluble penetrate body tissues and exhibit large distribution volumes.

Renal insufficiency frequently alters drug distribution volume. Edema and ascites may increase the apparent volume of distribution of highly water-soluble or protein-bound drugs. Usual doses given to edematous patients may result in inadequately low plasma levels. Conversely, dehydration or muscle wasting usually decreases the apparent volume of distribution of water-soluble drugs. In these cases, usual doses may result in unexpectedly high plasma concentrations.

The alteration of plasma protein binding in patients with renal insufficiency has an important effect on the volume of distribution of a drug, the quantity of free drug available for action, and the degree to which the agent can be excreted by the liver or kidneys. Protein-bound drugs attach reversibly to either albumin or glycoprotein in plasma. Organic acids often bind to a single binding site, whereas organic bases probably have multiple sites of attachment (5). The binding of many acidic drugs is decreased in renal failure. On the other hand, binding of organic bases is less affected by uremia (5).

Reduced plasma protein binding in uremic patients has been attributed to a combination of decreased serum albumin concentration and a reduction in albumin affinity for the drug. Affinity may be influenced by uremia-induced changes in the structural orientation of the albumin molecule or by the accumulation of endogenous inhibitors of protein binding that compete with drugs for their binding sites.

The therapeutic consequences of impaired plasma protein binding in uremia are important because the unbound fraction of several acidic drugs (e.g., salicylate, phenytoin) may be substantially increased. Serious toxicity can occur if the total plasma concentration is pushed into the therapeutic range by increasing the dose. For such drugs, total and unbound plasma concentrations should be measured.

Predicting the clinical consequences of altered protein binding in uremia is difficult. Although decreased binding results in more free drug being available at the site of drug action or toxicity, the distribution volume may be increased, producing lower plasma concentrations after a given dose. Because more unbound drug is available for metabolism and excretion, the half-life of the drug in the body may be decreased.

Metabolism

Renal failure substantially affects drug biotransformation. Reduction and hydrolysis reactions are generally slowed. Glucuronidation, sulfated conjugation, and microsomal oxidation usually occur at normal rates in patients with uremia (6).

Many active or toxic drug metabolites depend on renal function for elimination. The high incidence of adverse drug reactions seen in patients with renal failure may be explained in part by the accumulation of active metabolites (7).

Renal Excretion

The renal excretion of drugs depends on glomerular filtration and renal tubular secretion and reabsorption. The glomerular elimination of drugs also depends on the molecular size and protein binding of the agent. Although protein binding decreases the filtration of drugs, it may increase the amount that the renal tubule secretes. When glomerular filtration is impaired by renal disease, the clearance of drugs that are eliminated primarily by this mechanism will be decreased and the plasma half-life of the drugs prolonged.

Although we do not clinically measure tubular function, the secretion of drugs eliminated by active transport systems in the renal tubule also will be affected in patients with renal disease. Thus, as the rate of creatinine clearance decreases, drugs dependent on renal tubular secretion for elimination will be excreted more slowly. Furthermore, because the proximal tubular secretion of some agents is carrier mediated and capacity limited, concurrent use of multiple drugs eliminated by renal tubular secretion may saturate the transport system.

Pharmacokinetics

The term *pharmacokinetics* describes the time courses of drugs in the body. Models explain the absorption, distribution, metabolism, and excretion of drugs and their metabolites (1). After administration of the drug, an initial, high plasma concentration is followed by a rapid decrease in the drug level, which occurs as the drug is distributed from the plasma into the extravascular space. Concurrent with and following the distribution phase, the drug is eliminated at a slower rate. During the elimination phase, drug concentrations in plasma are in equilibrium with concentrations in body tissues.

Useful pharmacokinetic parameters may be developed using graphs of plasma drug concentrations after a dose is given. The rate and amount of drug absorption, the extent of distribution, and the rate of elimination may be measured. By comparing pharmacokinetic data from patients with normal renal function with those from patients with renal insufficiency, rational drug dosimetry may be determined for patients with impaired renal function. The tables in this guide use specific pharmacokinetic information; however, for many drugs for which data were inadequate or conflicting, the recommendations are based on the authors' judgments.

Dosimetry in Renal Disease

A rational approach to drug dosing in patients with renal impairment begins with a thorough history and physical examination. Particularly important is the history of previous drug allergy or toxicity, the use of concurrently prescribed or nonprescription medications, and the ingestion of alcohol or other recreational drugs. Physical assessment should include estimating the extracellular fluid volume; the presence of edema, ascites, or dehydration alters drug dose. Body weight and height need to be measured; for obese patients, the ideal body weight should be calculated and drug doses estimated accordingly. Evidence of impaired excretory organ function should be sought. Stigmata of chronic liver disease are a clue that drug dose may need to be severely altered.

A specific diagnosis should be established before drug therapy is initiated. Patients with renal failure receive many concurrent medications, often without specific indications, so medication lists should be reviewed frequently. Many adverse drug effects can be avoided if fewer agents are used and if potential drug interactions are recognized.

Renal Function

When the necessity for drug therapy has been established, renal function should be measured. Because the rate of elimination of drugs excreted by the kidneys is proportional to the glomerular filtration rate (GFR), the serum creatinine or creatinine clearance should be used to estimate renal function. The Cockroft and Gault equation can be used to estimate the creatinine clearance (CLcr) as shown in the following formula (8):

$$\text{CLcr} = \frac{(140 - \text{age}) \times \text{ideal body weight in kg}}{72 \times \text{serum creatinine in mg/dL}} \times 0.85 \text{ (for women)}$$

For men, ideal body weight = 50.0 kg + 2.3 kg/in over 5 ft tall
For women, ideal body weight = 45.5 kg + 2.3 kg/in over 5 ft tall

Estimating GFR from the serum creatinine level assumes that renal function is stable and that the serum creatinine measurement is constant. With changing renal function, the serum creatinine level will no longer reflect the true clearance rate, and creatinine clearance should be measured with a timed urine collection, using the midpoint value. If oliguria is present, the creatinine clearance may be estimated at less than 10 mL/min.

The serum creatinine is a function of muscle mass as well as GFR. Serum creatinine measurements within the "normal" range are frequently used to establish the presence of "normal" renal function, an erroneous assumption that may cause serious overdose and toxic drug accumulation in elderly or debilitated patients with diminished muscle mass.

Acute Renal Failure

The drug dosing guidelines in this book are derived mostly from studies performed in patients with stable, chronic renal insufficiency; however, these recommendations are often extrapolated to seriously ill patients with acutely decreased renal function. Studies have shown that pharmacokinetic parameters in patients with acute renal failure may differ from those measured in patients with chronic renal failure (9). Specifically, the nonrenal clearance of drugs decreases with the duration of renal failure. The preservation of nonrenal clearance observed early in the course of acute renal failure suggests that drug dosing schemes extrapolated from individuals with stable chronic renal failure could result in ineffectively low drug concentrations. Early in the course of the patient's therapy, individualized pharmacokinetic dosing for patients with acute renal failure is essential.

Initial Dose

If the physical examination suggests that the extracellular fluid volume is normal, the initial drug dose for a patient with renal failure is the same as that for a patient with normal renal function; however, if substantial edema or ascites is present, a larger initial dose may be necessary. Conversely, dehydrated or severely debilitated patients may require smaller initial doses. The purpose of the initial dose is to produce a therapeutic plasma drug concentration rapidly. Subsequent doses may need to be decreased to maintain therapeutic levels below the toxic range.

When a loading dose is given, levels within the therapeutic range are rapidly achieved. If no loading dose is prescribed, three to four half-lives of the drug will pass before the plasma levels are at steady-state. A loading dose should always be considered when the half-life of a drug is particularly long in a patient with renal failure or when rapid attainment of therapeutic plasma levels is critical.

Maintenance Dose

After the initial drug dose, subsequent doses may need to be modified in patients with diminished renal function. When renal function has been measured and the drug dose for patients with normal renal function determined, the appropriate dose for patients with impaired renal function can be calculated. Dosage guidelines for patients with normal and impaired renal function are provided in the tables.

Drug Removal by Extracorporeal Techniques

The effects of hemodialysis, peritoneal dialysis, and continuous arteriovenous or venovenous hemofiltration on drug elimination are difficult to predict. Factors affecting drug removal include molecular weight, lipid solubility, the chemistry and surface area of the dialysis membrane, blood and dialysate flow rates, drug protein binding, and red-cell partitioning. During dialysis, intermittent changes in drug clearance disrupt the drug concentration equilibrium between the central and peripheral compartments. Redistribution from the deeper compartments into the vascular space results in a rebound of plasma drug concentrations following the dialysis treatment.

New techniques of extracorporeal circulation for the treatment of renal failure include continuous arteriovenous hemofiltration and continuous venovenous hemofiltration, which use convective blood purification and continuous hemofiltration dialysis, which in turn add a diffusive component. Clearances of small-molecular-weight drugs are greater at higher dialysate flow rates because the removal of these compounds is substantially influenced by diffusion. Conversely, the clearance of large-molecular-weight compounds depends primarily on convection. Some compounds may even bind to some of the membranes used for hemofiltration.

The removal of most drugs during continuous renal replacement therapies (CRRT) has not been studied. The large number of drugs that may be given, the many variations of CRRT used, and the relatively few patients treated with CRRT make it unlikely that drug disposition during CRRT will be studied systematically. In the dose-supplement column labeled "CRRT," the recommendations are based on actual observations, when such data exist. Unfortunately, the majority of these dosing recommendations rely on theoretical extrapolations because measurements of drug removal have not been published. Consequently, these dosing suggestions should be applied cautiously and with the knowledge that they are estimates. When appropriate pharmacokinetic parameters are known, reasonable approximations can be made. This section outlines the assumptions that led to dosing estimates during CRRT.

Molecular weight was an important theoretical determinant of drug removal by CRRT. Larger molecular weight decreases drug diffusion through artificial membranes; however, high flux membranes and blood-pump driven filtration have increased extraction efficiency and make drug molecular weight a less important factor. In addition, blood pumping increases the transmembrane pressure, resulting in substantial drug removal by convection. Large molecular weight decreases diffusive drug transport more than convective drug transport. In addition, blood pumping increases the volume of blood passing through the filter, which further increases drug removal and lessens the importance of molecular size as a determinant of the amount of drug passing through the membrane. For drugs smaller than 1500 daltons, removal from the circulation is not substantially influenced by molecular size when high-flux membranes and blood pumping are used for CRRT.

The volume of distribution of a drug reflects its tissue binding. A large volume of distribution, arbitrarily defined as more than 0.7 L/kg, indicates a highly tissue-bound drug. Most of the compound is not accessible to the extracorporeal circulation for removal. The larger the volume of distribution, the less likely the drug will reach the CRRT filter. Even if extraction across the CRRT device is 100%, removal by CRRT is clinically insignificant because most of the drug in the body remains tissue bound.

Drug binding to serum proteins decreases drug removal by CRRT. Only unbound drug is available for pharmacologic activity, metabolism, excretion, and elimination by CRRT. The percent of unbound drug removed by CRRT also is influenced by the drug's molecular weight and distribution volume. A small solute with a small volume of distribution that is 70% protein bound results in 30% of the drug unbound in plasma. Its removal by CRRT may be substantial. Alternatively, a drug that is only 10% protein bound but which has a large volume of distribution will not be removed during CRRT, despite the large unbound fraction. This drug is present in the tissues rather than in the plasma entering the extracorporeal circuit.

Of the three drug factors that influence removal by CRRT, volume of distribution is the most important, followed by binding to serum proteins, and then molecular size.

When continuous hemofiltration occurs by spontaneous blood flow with no extracorporeal blood pumping, the CRRT-generated ultrafiltration rate is 10-15 mL/min. This value corresponds to an equivalent GFR when compared with native renal function. When blood pumps are used, ultrafiltration rates increase to 20-30 mL/min; thus, continuous hemofiltration results in drug clearance similar to a GFR of 10-30 mL/min. If continuous dialysis is used, the diffusive component may add another 15-20 mL/min of drug clearance, depending on the dialysate flow rate and the membrane flux. CRRT, therefore, functions at a drug filtration rate of 10-50 mL/min, depending on the blood flow rate, the membrane flux, and the use of dialysate.

In summary, dosing recommendations during CRRT are based on actual clearance data when available. When measurements are not available, estimates of drug clearance are made based on protein binding and volume of distribution. A volume of distribution 0.7 L/kg is considered influential in decreasing CRRT drug removal. A protein binding of greater than 80% suggests that much of the drug will not be removed convectively or by diffusion. Continuous renal replacement therapies are similar to high-flux dialysis in total solute clearance and correspond to a GFR of 10-50 mL/min.

Therapeutic Drug Monitoring

Clinical application of pharmacokinetic principles to individualize dosage regimens is called *therapeutic drug monitoring*. The recently developed sensitive and specific assays for plasma drug concentrations and inexpensive computer hardware and software are alternatives to drug dosing by trial and error. Appropriate pharmacokinetic application of drug-level measurements can improve patient care at a decreased cost (10-12).

Measurement of plasma drug concentrations may help in assessing a particular drug-dosing regimen when the relationship between drug levels and efficacy or toxicity has been established. These concentrations are particularly important for drugs with a narrow range between therapeutic and toxic levels and for drugs whose pharmacologic effects are not readily measured. Plasma-level monitoring, however, has little value for drugs with an effect that is easily measured or irreversible. For example, antihypertensive efficacy parallels plasma drug concentrations but can be easily determined by monitoring blood pressure and heart rate.

Generally, three or four doses of the drug should be given before plasma levels are measured to ensure that steady-state concentrations have been established. For some drugs, both maximum and minimum concentrations are relevant. Peak levels are most meaningful when measured after rapid drug distribution has occurred. For example, aminoglycoside peak concentrations usually are measured 30 minutes after the infusion. Minimum plasma drug concentrations should be measured immediately before the next dose is given. Trough levels are more reliable measurements of drug elimination and reflect more closely potential drug accumulation in patients with renal failure.

Many institutions offer formal dosing services. Although they are often pharmacy based, these services should be multidisciplinary and should include the primary physician and subspecialty consultants.

Based on the patient's clinical state, concurrent medications, blood level pharmacokinetics, and response to therapy, consultants provide advice on drug dose, interval, route of administration, and timing of plasma levels. Final recommendations often include literature references, adverse drug effects, and potential drug interactions (12).

Adverse Drug Reactions

Despite careful consideration of uremia-induced changes in drug disposition, adverse drug responses remain common in patients with impaired renal function (13,14). Some toxicity may be eliminated by avoiding drugs known to cause adverse events, which can result from direct toxicity of the drug or its metabolites, poor efficacy of the drug in decreased renal function, or production of an increased metabolic load that diseased kidneys cannot excrete.

A drug's potential for direct renal toxicity is particularly important in patients with reduced renal function. Even a mild renal injury in a patient with diminished renal reserve may be catastrophic. Drugs may precipitate direct renal tubule toxicity, obstructive uropathy, glomerulonephritis, interstitial nephritis, and disturbances of sodium and water and acid-base balance. The accumulation of active or toxic metabolites may lead to unexpected drug reactions. Acute onset of any unexplained symptoms should alert clinicians to a possible adverse drug effect.

Patients with renal failure are heterogeneous, and their responses to drug therapy are variable. Dosage nomograms, dosage tables, and computer-assisted dosing recommendations should not be taken as a fixed approach but rather as an initial attempt to arrive at an effective dose regime. The authors have included the dose of most drugs used for patients with normal renal function. These doses vary with the specific needs of individual patients, as does appropriate adjustment for patients with renal failure. In addition, specific supplementary doses for patients undergoing hemodialysis, continuous ambulatory peritoneal dialysis, and continuous arteriovenous hemofiltration are provided. Physicians using sound clinical judgment in caring for patients with renal disease should evaluate each situation, choose a drug regimen based on all factors, and continually re-evaluate response to therapy.

Pharmacokinetic studies have led to the development of inclusive nomograms and tables of drug disposition and dosimetry for patients with renal impairment. The tables in this book contain dose recommendations based on the most current information available.

References

1. **Wagner JG.** Fundamentals of Clinical Pharmacokinetics. Hamilton, Illinois: Drug Intelligence Publications, Inc.; 1975:337-58.

2. **Anderson RJ, Gambertoglio JG, Schrier RW.** Clinical Use of Drugs in Renal Failure. Springfield, Illinois: Charles C. Thomas; 1976.

3. **Hurwitz A.** Antacid therapy and drug kinetics. Clin Pharmacokinet. 1977;2:269-80.

4. **Craig R, Murphy T, Gibson TP.** Kinetic analysis of D-xylose absorption in normal subjects and in patients with chronic renal insufficiency. J Lab Clin Med. 1983;101:496-506.

5. **Reidenberg MM.** The binding of drugs to plasma proteins and the interpretation of measurements of plasma concentration of drugs in patients with poor renal function. Am J Med. 1977;62:482-5.

6. **Reidenberg MM.** The biotransformation of drugs in renal failure. Am J Med. 1977;62:482-5.

7. **Verbeeck RK, Branch RA, Wilkinson GR.** Drug metabolites in renal failure: pharmacokinetic and clinical implications. Clin Pharmacokinet. 1981;6:329-45.

8. **Cockroft DW, Gault MH.** Prediction of creatinine clearance from serum creatinine. Nephron. 1976;16:31-41.

9. **Macias WL, Mueller BA, Scarim SK.** Vancomycin pharmacokinetics in acute renal failure: preservation of nonrenal clearance. Clin Phamacol Ther. 1991;50:688-94.

10. **Bollish SJ, Kelly WN, Miller DE, Timmons RG.** Establishing and aminoglycoside pharmacokinetic service in a community hospital. Am J Hosp Pharm. 1981;38:73-6.

11. **Elenbaas RM, Payne VW, Bauman JL.** Influence of clinical pharmacist consultations on the use of drug blood level tests. Am J Hosp Pharm. 1980;37:61-4.

12. **Aronoff GR, Abel SR.** Principles of administering drugs to patients with renal failure. In: Brenner BM, Stein JH, eds. Contemporary Issues in Nephrology. New York: Churchill-Livingstone. 1986.

13. **Jick H.** Adverse drug effects in relation to renal function. Am J Med. 1977;62:514-7.

14. **Smith JW, Seidl LG, Cluff LE.** Studies on the epidemiology of adverse drug reaction: V. Clinical factors influencing susceptibility. Ann Intern Med. 1966;65:629-40.

Use of the Tables

Drugs in this book are listed in alphabetical order by generic name under subdivisions based on similarity of structure and pharmacologic action. For example, penicillins, cephalosporins, and aminoglycosides are grouped together as antibiotics.

Toxicity and Notes

Nephrotoxicity or systemic adverse effects and information specifically related to patients with renal disease are listed just under the generic drug name. Remarks common to all members of a class or group of drugs are listed under the name of the drug class and generally apply to each drug in the group.

Major Excretion Route

The second column lists the percentage of total drug excreted unchanged in the urine for patients with normal renal function. For some drugs, the second column gives the major route of elimination or metabolism. Drugs that are extensively metabolized by the liver or extracted during their initial circulation through the liver after gastrointestinal absorption have complex pharmacokinetics. For these drugs, the half-life given is for disappearance of active drug after it has reached the general circulation. In patients with hepatic dysfunction, the percentage of an administered dose metabolized by the "first pass" effect may be reduced. For the tables, it is assumed that liver function is normal and that other drugs that alter hepatic metabolism are not being given.

Pharmacokinetic Variables

Dosage adjustments for renal failure depend on knowledge of normal drug disposition. Pharmacokinetic variables in normal subjects are given in the tables. These variables include the major route of drug elimination by either excretion or metabolism, the plasma or biologic half-life for patients with normal renal function and for end-stage renal disease, the extent of drug binding to plasma proteins, and the apparent volume of distribution. The volume of distribution and half-life given should be considered when estimating blood levels after dosage, finding the proper maintenance regimen, and deciding the likelihood of drug removal by dialysis. As outlined above, the complex pharmacokinetics and variability of drug disposition in patients with renal failure cannot be adequately described by these simple parameters.

Dosage for Normal Renal Function

After the pharmacokinetic variables, drug doses sometimes given to patients with normal renal function are listed. These recommendations are meant only as a guide and do not imply efficacy of a listed dosage.

Dosage Adjustment for Renal Failure

A loading dose should be considered when the half-life of a drug is particularly long in patients with impaired renal function. When the physical examination suggests that the extracellular fluid volume is normal, the loading dose of a drug given to a patient with renal insufficiency is the same as the initial dose given to a patient with normal renal function. Initial doses for most drugs that require loading are already known; however, the loading dose may be calculated using the formula

$$\text{Loading Dose} = \text{Vd (L/kg)} \times \text{Wt (kg)} \times \text{Cp (mg/L)}$$

where
    Vd = volume of distribution of the drug,
    Wt = patient's ideal body weight, and
    Cp = desired plasma drug level.

Patients with substantial edema or ascites may require a somewhat larger loading dose, whereas patients who are dehydrated or debilitated should receive smaller initial drug doses.

To adjust the maintenance dosage in patients with renal insufficiency, the intervals between individual doses can be lengthened (interval extension method), keeping the dose size normal. The calculated dose interval should be rounded to a convenient time schedule. This method is particularly useful for drugs with wide therapeutic ranges and long plasma half-lives in patients with renal impairment. Interval lengthening will result in wide swings of the plasma drug concentrations from peak to trough levels. If the range between the therapeutic and toxic levels is too narrow, either toxic or subtherapeutic plasma concentrations may result.

Alternatively, the size of the individual doses can be reduced, keeping the interval between doses normal. Decreasing the individual doses reduces the difference between peak and trough plasma concentrations. This effect is important for drugs with narrow therapeutic ranges and short plasma half-lives in patients with renal impairment and is recommended for drugs for which a relatively constant blood level is desired. The reduced dose should be rounded to a convenient value.

In the tables, the preferred method for dosage adjustment is included for each drug. Dose reduction is indicated by "D" and interval extension by "I." After the recommended method for dosage adjustment, recommendations are given for levels of renal function, as estimated by the glomerular filtration rate. For the dose-reduction method, the percentage of the usual dose that should be given at the normal dose interval is shown. When the interval extension method is recommended, the number of hours between doses of normal size is given.

No controlled clinical trials have been performed to establish the efficacy of the two methods for drug-dose alteration in patients with renal insufficiency. Prolonging the dose interval is often more convenient and less expensive. When the dose interval can safely be lengthened beyond 24 hours, extended parenteral therapy may be completed without prolonged hospitalization. In patients requiring chronic hemodialysis, many drugs need to be given only at the end of the dialysis treatment. Furthermore, compliance with any drug regimen may be better when fewer doses can be taken at convenient times.

In practice, a combination of interval prolongation and dose-size reduction is often effective and convenient. The recommendations given for aminoglycosides are an attempt to combine these considerations by decreasing the individual aminoglycoside doses and by increasing the dosage interval.

Dialysis Adjustment

The effect of standard clinical treatment on drug removal is shown for hemodialysis (Hemo), chronic ambulatory peritoneal dialysis (CAPD), and continuous renal replacement therapy (CRRT). When known, specific recommendations for dose adjustment are given. Some drugs that have high dialysis clearance do not require supplemental doses after dialysis if the amount of drug removed is not sufficient, as would be the case if the volume of distribution is large. To simplify dosimetry and to ensure efficacy when information about dialysis loss is not available, maintenance doses of most drugs should be given after dialysis. Peritonitis is a major complication of CAPD, and treatment usually involves intraperitoneal administration of antibiotics. For some drugs, sophisticated pharmacokinetic studies are available, whereas for others drugs, use is still based on empirical dosage recommendations. In general, there is excellent drug absorption after intraperitoneal administration of common antibiotics. Factors favoring absorption include inflamed membranes and concentration gradients. For drugs such as aminoglycosides, cephalosporins, and penicillins, the drug levels in peritoneal fluid after intravenous or oral administration are inconsistent.

The following abbreviations are used in the tables:

BUN—blood urea nitrogen; Ca^{++}—factor IV calcium; CAPD—chronic ambulatory peritoneal dialysis; CAVH—continuous arteriovenous or venovenous hemofiltration; CNS—central nervous system; D—dosage reduction method; ESRD—end-stage renal disease; GFR—glomerular filtration rate; Hemo—hemodialysis; I—interval extension method; K^+—potassium; Mg^{++}—magnesium; Na^+—sodium; NSAIDs—nonsteroidal anti-inflammatory drugs; PO4—phosphate radical; SIADH—syndrome of inappropriate secretion of antidiuretic hormone; $T_{1/2}$—biologic half-life; UTI—urinary tract infection; Vd—volume of distribution of the drug.

Analgesics

Hepatic metabolism eliminates most commonly used analgesics. They require little dose reduction for patients with renal insufficiency. Saturable, nonlinear excretion complicates salicylate elimination kinetics. Because of the hemorrhagic diathesis in patients with severe renal failure and the variability of salicylate elimination, avoid large doses of aspirin in patients with severe renal failure. Narcotic analgesics produce sedation that may be more profound in patients with renal insufficiency. Carefully titrate the doses of these drugs and use the smallest effective dose for the shortest possible time.

Meperidine requires special care. The primary metabolite, normeperidine, has little analgesic effect, accumulates in patients with renal failure, and may decrease the seizure threshold. Reports document similar less-frequent effects with morphine and its metabolite normorphine. Although meperidine and morphine can be used in patients with severe renal failure, avoid repetitive doses.

Analgesics

Drug, Toxicity Notes	Percent Excreted Unchanged (%)	Half-Life (Normal/ESRD) (h)	Plasma Protein Binding (%)	Volume of Distribution (L/kg)	Dose for Normal Renal Function	Method	Adjustment for Renal Failure GFR, mL/min >50	10-50	<10	Supplement for Dialysis
Narcotics and Narcotic Antagonists										
Alfentanil	Hepatic	1-3/Unknown	88-95	0.3-1	Anesthetic induction 8-40 µg/kg	D	100%	100%	100%	Hemo: Not applicable CAPD: Not applicable CAVH: Not applicable
Butorphanol	Hepatic	2-4/No data	80	9-11	2 mg q3-4h	D	100%	75%	50%	Hemo: No data CAPD: No data CAVH: Not applicable
Codeine	Hepatic	2.5-3.5/No data	7	3-4	30-60 mg q4-6h	D	100%	75%	50%	Hemo: No data CAPD: No data CAVH: Dose for GFR 10-50
Fentanyl	Hepatic	2-7/No data	80-84	2-4	Anesthetic induction (individualized)	D	100%	75%	50%	Hemo: Not applicable CAPD: Not applicable CAVH: Not applicable
Meperidine	Hepatic	2-7/7-32	70	4-5	50-100 mg q3-4h	D	100%	75%	50%	Hemo: Avoid CAPD: Avoid CAVH: Avoid
Normeperidine, an active metabolite, accumulates in ESRD and may cause seizures. Protein binding is reduced in ESRD. 20-25% excreted unchanged in acidic urine.										
Methadone	Hepatic	13-58/No data	60-90	3-6	2.5-10 mg q6-8h	D	100%	100%	50-75%	Hemo: None CAPD: None CAVH: Not applicable

Drug	Route of Metabolism	Half-life Normal/ESRD	% Protein Binding	Vd	Dose for Normal Renal Function	Method	GFR >50	GFR 10-50	GFR <10	Dialysis
Morphine	Hepatic	1-4/Unchanged	20-30	3.5	20-25 mg q4h	D	100%	75%	50%	Hemo: None CAPD: No data CAVH: Dose for GFR 10-50
Increased sensitivity to drug effect in ESRD.										
Naloxone	Hepatic	1.0-1.5/No data	54	3	2 mg IV	D	100%	100%	100%	Hemo: Not applicable CAPD: Not applicable CAVH: Dose for GFR 10-50
Pentazocine	Hepatic	2-5/No data	50-75	5	50 mg q4h	D	100%	75%	50%	Hemo: None CAPD: No data CAVH: Dose for GFR 10-50
Propoxyphene	Hepatic	9-15/12-20	78	16	65 mg po q6-8h	D	100%	100%	Avoid	Hemo: Avoid CAPD: Avoid CAVH: Not applicable
Active metabolite norpropoxyphene accumulates in ESRD.										
Sufentanil	Hepatic	2-5/Unchanged	92	2-3	Anesthetic induction (individualized)	D	100%	100%	100%	Hemo: Not applicable CAPD: Not applicable CAVH: Not applicable

Non-Narcotics

Drug	Route of Metabolism	Half-life Normal/ESRD	% Protein Binding	Vd	Dose for Normal Renal Function	Method	GFR >50	GFR 10-50	GFR <10	Dialysis
Acetaminophen	Hepatic	2/2	20-30	1-2	650 mg q4h	I	q4h	q6h	q8h	Hemo: None CAPD: None CAVH: Dose for GFR 10-50
Overdose may be nephrotoxic. Drug is major metabolite of phenacetin.										
Aspirin (USP)	Hepatic (renal)	2-3/Unchanged	80-90	0.1-0.2	650 mg q4h	I	q4h	q4-6h	Avoid	Hemo: Dose after dialysis CAPD: None CAVH: Dose for GFR 10-50

For definitions of the abbreviations used in the tables, see page 16.

19

Antihypertensive and Cardiovascular Agents

Hypertension and coronary heart disease occur frequently in patients with impaired renal function. Antihypertensive and cardiovascular agents are the most commonly prescribed drugs in patients with renal disease. Narrow therapeutic range and individual variability in drug response complicate the use of these drugs. As indicated in the table, some of these drugs or their metabolites accumulate in patients with renal insufficiency. Abnormalities of drug binding to plasma proteins increase free drug at receptor sites, enhancing both drug efficacy and toxicity.

The relationship between renal drug elimination and the cardiovascular system is well established. Drugs may alter their own elimination rate or their effect on the kidneys by improving cardiac output and effective renal blood flow. For example, patients with decompensated congestive heart failure may be resistant to diuretics. If natriuresis can be initiated, the subsequent improvement in cardiovascular function can increase response to the diuretic. Thus, the effect of cardiovascular drugs may also vary for individual patients as cardiac function changes.

The use of antiarrhythmic agents requires particular care. Because toxicity may appear as the arrhythmia that the drug is intended to correct, recognition of toxicity may be delayed. Inappropriate increases in antiarrhythmic dose may be fatal. Monitoring other electrocardiographic evidence of toxicity (e.g., prolonged QT interval, widening of the QRS complex) may be essential to proper diagnosis.

Procainamide presents particular difficulty in patients with renal dysfunction. Its elimination is slowed by renal failure; the excretion of its primary metabolite, *N*-acetyl procainamide, depends on kidney function; and the parent drug and the metabolite appear to have different antiarrhythmic spectra and elimination rates. Avoiding procainamide in patients with renal impairment would seem prudent, but this approach is often not practical. Careful monitoring is essential, and measurement of drug and metabolite levels may be helpful.

The kidney excretes many antihypertensive agents. The wide variability of drug response makes it necessary that the response of blood pressure to dose be monitored for individual patients. Steady-state drug levels are usually not achieved until after the drug has been given for at least three or four half-lives. The data in the table may be useful in predicting the best time for changing the dose during the titration process.

Diuretics remain an essential part of most antihypertensive therapy. They can be grouped into two categories based on their clinical use. The potassium-sparing drugs (amiloride, spironolactone, and triamterene) may produce hyperkalemia in patients with creatinine clearances below 30 mL/min and should be avoided in these patients. The remaining diuretics are organic acids and need to reach the tubular lumen to be active. In patients with impaired renal function, endogenous organic acids accumulate and compete with diuretics for secretion into the tubular lumen. Consequently, as renal function decreases, larger doses of diuretics are required. As glomerular filtration falls, the thiazides become ineffective; however, large doses of the loop diuretics (furosemide, bumetanide, and ethacrynic acid) may still produce diuresis. In patients with renal insufficiency, diuretic-induced dehydration may result in a further loss of renal function. Unless patients require diuresis for substantial peripheral edema or congestive heart failure, hypertension in patients with decreased renal function should be managed to avoid unnecessary volume contraction.

Each of the antihypertensive drugs listed in the table can be toxic. In general, the adverse effects are related to pharmacologic effect and can be avoided by careful dose titration. The development of newer, effective antihypertensive agents allows more individualized pharmacotherapy. In choosing an antihypertensive agent, one should understand the altered homeostatic mechanisms in patients with impaired renal function.

When blood pressure is appropriately lowered in hypertensive patients with renal insufficiency, a transient decrease in renal function may occur. As hypertensive microvascular changes improve, renal function should increase. In some cases, dialysis may be needed temporarily. If renal function decreases with antihypertensive therapy and does not improve, drug-related nephrotoxicity or another potentially reversible cause should be considered.

The choice of cardiac glycosides in patients with renal insufficiency is controversial. The kidneys excrete digoxin. Reduce digoxin doses substantially for patients with even modest decreases in renal function. Because the liver excretes digitoxin, only patients with severe renal impairment require dosage reduction; however, digitoxin's long half-life makes toxicity with this drug potentially more serious. Both drugs have a smaller volume of distribution in patients with renal insufficiency, making calculation of the appropriate loading dose more difficult. When digitalization can be done gradually, give a small loading dose followed by reduced maintenance doses.

Antihypertensive and Cardiovascular Agents

Drug, Toxicity Notes	Percent Excreted Unchanged	Half-Life (Normal/ ESRD)	Plasma Protein Binding	Volume of Distribution	Dose for Normal Renal Function	Method	>50	10-50	<10	Supplement for Dialysis
								Adjustment for Renal Failure GFR, mL/min		
	%	h	%	L/kg						

Antihypertensive Drugs

Adrenergic and Serotoninergic Modulators
Blood pressure is the best guide to dose and interval.

Drug, Toxicity Notes	Percent Excreted Unchanged	Half-Life (Normal/ ESRD)	Plasma Protein Binding	Volume of Distribution	Dose for Normal Renal Function	Method	>50	10-50	<10	Supplement for Dialysis
Clonidine	45	6-23/39-42	20-40	3-6	0.1-0.6 mg bid	D	100%	100%	100%	Hemo: None CAPD: None CAVH: Dose for GFR 10-50
Rebound hypertension if drug is abruptly withdrawn. Tricyclic antidepressants decrease efficacy. Potentiates CNS depressant effects of alcohol, sedatives.										
Doxazosin	< 5	16-22/16-22	98	1.0-1.7	1-16 mg q24h	D	100%	100%	100%	Hemo: None CAPD: None CAVH: Dose for GFR 10-50
May produce profound first-dose hypotension. Titration of renal patients should begin from low doses.										
Guanabenz	< 5	12-14/No data	90	10-12	8-16 mg bid	D	100%	100%	100%	Hemo: No data CAPD: No data CAVH: Dose for GFR 10-50
Similar to clonidine.										
Guanadrel	30-40	4-10/19	20	11.5	10-50 mg bid	I	q12h	q12-24h	q24-48h	Hemo: No data CAPD: No data CAVH: Dose for GFR 10-50
Similar to guanethidine, but less diarrhea.										
Guanethidine	25-50	120-140/No data	< 5	No data	10-100 mg q24h	I	q24h	q24h	q24-36h	Hemo: No data CAPD: No data CAVH: Avoid
Tricyclic antidepressants decrease efficacy. Causes orthostatic hypotension, diarrhea.										

Drug	% Excreted	Half-life (Normal/ESRD)	Protein Binding (%)	Dose	Method	GFR >50	GFR 10-50	GFR <10	Supplement
Guanfacine	24-37	12-23/15-25	65	1-2 mg q24h	D	100%	100%	100%	Hemo: None CAPD: None CAVH: Dose for GFR 10-50
Ketanserin	<2	14-19/25-35	95	40 mg bid	D	100%	100%	100%	Hemo: None CAPD: None CAVH: Dose for GFR 10-50
Methyldopa	25-40	1.5-6.0/6-16	<15	250-500 mg tid	I	q8h	q8-12h	q12-24h	Hemo: 250 mg CAPD: None CAVH: Dose for GFR 10-50
Prazosin	<5	2-3/2-3	97	1-15 mg bid	D	100%	100%	100%	Hemo: None CAPD: None CAVH: Dose for GFR 10-50
Reserpine	<1	46-168/87-323	96	0.05-0.25 mg q24h	D	100%	100%	Avoid	Hemo: None CAPD: None CAVH: Dose for GFR 10-50
Terazosin	20-30	9-12/8-12	90-94	1-20 mg q24h	D	100%	100%	100%	Hemo: No data CAPD: No data CAVH: Dose for GFR 10-50

Guanfacine: Similar to clonidine, but milder.

Ketanserin: Serotonin receptor antagonist; protein binding decreased in uremia.

Methyldopa: Orthostatic hypotension. Retroperitoneal fibrosis. Elevates serum creatinine by acting as a chromogen. Active metabolites with long half-life.

Prazosin: May produce profound first-dose hypotension. Titration of renal patients should begin from low doses.

Reserpine: Excessive sedation. Gastrointestinal bleeding.

Terazosin: Similar to prazosin.

Angiotensin-II–Receptor Antagonists

Blood pressure is the best guide to dose and interval. Hypotensive effects magnified by natriuretic agents or sodium depletion. Can cause hyperkalemia, metabolic acidosis. Acute renal dysfunction with bilateral or transplant renal artery stenosis, low renal perfusion pressure. Dry cough in 5-10%.

Drug	% Excreted	Half-life (Normal/ESRD)	Protein Binding (%)	Dose	Method	GFR >50	GFR 10-50	GFR <10	Supplement
Losartan	10-15	3/4-6	30	50 mg q12h	D	100%	100%	100%	Hemo: No data CAPD: No data CAVH: Dose for GFR 10-50

For definitions of the abbreviations used in the tables, see page 16.

Antihypertensive and Cardiovascular Agents (Continued)

Drug, Toxicity Notes	Percent Excreted Unchanged	Half-Life (Normal/ ESRD)	Plasma Protein Binding	Volume of Distribution	Dose for Normal Renal Function	Method	Adjustment for Renal Failure GFR, mL/min >50	10-50	<10	Supplement for Dialysis
	%	h	%	L/kg						

Antihypertensive Drugs (Continued)

Angiotensin-Converting–Enzyme Inhibitors

Blood pressure is the best guide to dose and interval. Hypotensive effects magnified by natriuretic agents or sodium depletion. Can cause hyperkalemia, metabolic acidosis. Acute renal dysfunction with bilateral or transplant renal artery stenosis, low renal perfusion pressure. Dry cough in 5–10%.

Drug, Toxicity Notes	Percent Excreted Unchanged	Half-Life (Normal/ ESRD)	Plasma Protein Binding	Volume of Distribution	Dose for Normal Renal Function	Method	>50	10-50	<10	Supplement for Dialysis
Benazepril	20	22/30	95	0.15	10 mg q24h	D	100%	50-75%	25-50%	Hemo: None CAPD: None CAVH: Dose for GFR 10-50
Captopril	30-40	2-3/21-32	25-30	0.7-3	25 mg q8h	D,I	100% q8-12h	75% q12-18h	50% q24h	Hemo: 25-30% CAPD: None CAVH: Dose for GFR 10-50
Rare proteinuria, nephrotic syndrome, dysgeusia, granulocytopenia. Increases serum digoxin levels.										
Cilazapril	80-90	40-50/> 60	No data	0.5-0.8	1.25 mg q24h	D,I	75% q24h	50% q24-48h	10-25% q72h	Hemo: None CAPD: None CAVH: Dose for GFR 10-50
Cilazaprilat, the active moiety formed in liver.										
Enalapril	43	11-24/34-60	50-60	No data	5-10 mg q12h	D	100%	75-100%	50%	Hemo: 20-25% CAPD: None CAVH: Dose for GFR 10-50
Enalaprilat, the active moiety formed in liver.										
Fosinopril	9-16	12/14-32	95	0.15	10 mg q24h	D	100%	100%	75-100%	Hemo: None CAPD: None CAVH: Dose for GFR 10-50
Fosinoprilat, the active moiety formed in liver. Drug less likely than other angiotensin-converting enzyme inhibitors to accumulate in renal failure.										

Drug					Method	GFR >50	GFR 10-50	GFR <10	Supplement for Dialysis
Lisinopril	80-90	30/40-50	0-10	0.13-0.15	5-10 mg q24h	D	100%	50-75%	25-50%	Hemo: 20% CAPD: None CAVH: Dose for GFR 10-50
Lysine analog of a pharmacologically active enalapril metabolite.									
Pentopril	80-90	2-3/10-14	60	0.8	125 mg q24h	D	100%	50-75%	50%	Hemo: No data CAPD: No data CAVH: Dose for GFR 10-50
Perindopril	<10	5/27	20	0.6-0.8	2 mg q24h	D	100%	75%	50%	Hemo: 25-50% CAPD: No data CAVH: Dose for GFR 10-50
Quinapril	30	1-2/6-15	97	1.5	10-20 mg q24h	D	100%	75-100%	75%	Hemo: 25% CAPD: None CAVH: Dose for GFR 10-50
Ramipril	10-21	5-8/15	55-70	1.2	10-20 mg q24h	D	100%	50-75%	25-50%	Hemo: 20% CAPD: None CAVH: Dose for GFR 10-50

Beta-Blockers

Blood pressure is the best guide to dose and interval. Hyperkalemia in ESRD.

Drug					Method	GFR >50	GFR 10-50	GFR <10	Supplement for Dialysis
Acebutolol	55	7-9?/7	20	1.2	400-600 mg q24h or bid	D	100%	50%	30-50%	Hemo: None CAPD: None CAVH: Dose for GFR 10-50
Active metabolites with long half-life.									
Atenolol	>90	6.7/15-35	3	1.1	50-100 mg q24h	D,I	100% q24h	50% q48h	30-50% q96h	Hemo: 25-50 mg CAPD: None CAVH: Dose for GFR 10-50
Accumulates in ESRD.									
Betaxolol	80-90	15-20/30-35	45-60	5-10	20 mg q24h	D	100%	100%	50%	Hemo: None CAPD: None CAVH: Dose for GFR 10-50

For definitions of the abbreviations used in the tables, see page 16.

Antihypertensive and Cardiovascular Agents (Continued)

Drug, Toxicity Notes	Percent Excreted Unchanged	Half-Life (Normal/ESRD)	Plasma Protein Binding	Volume of Distribution	Dose for Normal Renal Function	Adjustment for Renal Failure				Supplement for Dialysis
						Method	GFR, mL/min			
							>50	10-50	<10	
	%	h	%	L/kg						
Antihypertensive Drugs (Continued)										
Beta-Blockers (Continued)										
Bisoprolol	50	9-13/18-24	30-35	3	10 mg q24h	D	100%	75%	50%	Hemo: No data CAPD: No data CAVH: Dose for GFR 10-50
Bopindolol	< 10	4-10/Unchanged	No data	2-3	1-4 mg q24h	D	100%	100%	100%	Hemo: None CAPD: None CAVH: Dose for GFR 10-50
Carteolol	> 50	7/33	20-30	4.0	0.5-10 mg q24h	D	100%	50%	25%	Hemo: No data CAPD: None CAVH: Dose for GFR 10-50
Carvedilol	< 2	5-8/5-8	95	1-2	25-50 mg q12-24h	D	100%	100%	100%	Hemo: None CAPD: None CAVH: Dose for GFR 10-50
Celiprolol	10	4-5/5	No data	No data	200 mg q24h	D	100%	100%	75%	Hemo: No data CAPD: None CAVH: Dose for GFR 10-50
Dilevalol	< 5	8-12/19-30	75	25	200-400 mg bid	D	100%	100%	100%	Hemo: None CAPD: None CAVH: No data

Drug				Dose					
Esmolol	<10	7-15 min/Unchanged	No data	No data		D	100%	100%	100%	Hemo: None CAPD: None CAVH: No data
Active metabolite retained in renal failure.									
Labetalol	<5	3-9/Unchanged	50	5.6	200-600 mg bid	D	100%	100%	100%	Hemo: None CAPD: None CAVH: Dose for GFR 10-50
Metoprolol	5	3.5/2.5-4.5	8	5.5	50-100 mg bid	D	100%	100%	100%	Hemo: 50 mg CAPD: None CAVH: Dose for GFR 10-50
Nadolol	90	19/45	28	1.9	80-120 mg q24h	D	100%	50%	25%	Hemo: 40 mg CAPD: None CAVH: Dose for GFR 10-50
Penbutolol	<10	22/24	>95	No data	10-40 mg q24h	D	100%	100%	100%	Hemo: None CAPD: None CAVH: Dose for GFR 10-50
Pindolol	40	2.5-4.0/3-4	50	1.2	10-40 mg bid	D	100%	100%	100%	Hemo: None CAPD: None CAVH: Dose for GFR 10-50
Propranolol	<5	2-6/1-6	93	2.8	80-160 mg bid	D	100%	100%	100%	Hemo: None CAPD: None CAVH: Dose for GFR 10-50
Bioavailability may increase in ESRD. Metabolites may cause increased bilirubin by assay interference in ESRD.									
Sotalol	60	7.5-15.0/56	<1	1.3	160 mg q24h	D	100%	30%	15-30%	Hemo: 80 mg CAPD: None CAVH: Dose for GFR 10-50
Hypoglycemia reported in ESRD.									
Timolol	15	2.7/4.0	60	1.7	10-20 mg bid	D	100%	100%	100%	Hemo: None CAPD: None CAVH: Dose for GFR 10-50

For definitions of the abbreviations used in the tables, see page 16.

Antihypertensive and Cardiovascular Agents (Continued)

Drug, Toxicity Notes	Percent Excreted Unchanged	Half-Life (Normal/ ESRD)	Plasma Protein Binding	Volume of Distribution	Dose for Normal Renal Function	Method	Adjustment for Renal Failure GFR, mL/min >50	10-50	<10	Supplement for Dialysis
	%	h	%	L/kg						

Antihypertensive Drugs (Continued)

Vasodiliators
Blood pressure is the best guide to dose and interval.

Drug, Toxicity Notes	Percent Excreted Unchanged	Half-Life (Normal/ ESRD)	Plasma Protein Binding	Volume of Distribution	Dose for Normal Renal Function	Method	>50	10-50	<10	Supplement for Dialysis
Diazoxide Sodium and water retention.	50	17-31/30-60	> 90	0.2-0.3	150-300 mg IV bolus	D	100%	100%	100%	Hemo: None CAPD: None CAVH: Dose for GFR 10-50
Hydralazine Drug-induced lupus erythematosus.	25	2.0-4.5/7-16	87	0.5-0.9	25-50 mg tid	I	q8h	q8h	q8-16h	Hemo: None CAPD: None CAVH: Dose for GFR 10-50
Minoxidil Fluid retention, pericardial effusion.	15-20	2.8-4.2/Unchanged	0	2-3	5-30 mg bid	D	100%	100%	100%	Hemo: None CAPD: None CAVH: Dose for GFR 10-50
Nitroprusside	< 10	< 10 min/< 10 min	0	0.2	0.25-8.0 µg/kg/min by infusion	D	100%	100%	100%	Hemo: None CAPD: None CAVH: Dose for GFR 10-50

Toxic metabolite, thiocyanate, accumulates causing seizures, coma. Thiocyanate is hemodialyzable. Measure thiocyanate levels.

Cardiovascular Agents

Antiarrhythmic Agents

Blood levels most often the best guide to therapy. Half-life may be prolonged in heart failure or with reduced hepatic blood flow.

Adenosine	< 5	< 10 sec/Unchanged	0	No data	3-6 mg IV bolus	D	100%	100%	100%	Hemo: None CAPD: None CAVH: Dose for GFR 10-50
Amiodarone	< 5	14-120 d/Unchanged	96	70-140	800-2000 mg load then 200-600 mg q24h	D	100%	100%	100%	Hemo: None CAPD: None CAVH: Dose for GFR 10-50

Hepatotoxicity. Thyroid dysfunction. Peripheral neuropathy. Pulmonary fibrosis. Increased plasma digoxin.
Increases cyclosporine levels.

Bretylium Hypotension.	75	6.0-13.6/16-32	6	8.2	5-30 mg/kg load then 5-10 mg IV q6h	D	100%	25-50%	25%	Hemo: None CAPD: None CAVH: Dose for GFR 10-50
Cibenzoline	50-60	7/22	50	4-5	130-160 mg q12h	D,I	100% q12h	100% q12h	66% q24h	Hemo: None CAPD: None CAVH: Dose for GFR 10-50
Disopyramide	35-65	5-8/10-18	54-81	0.8-2.6	100-200 mg q6h	I	q8h	q12-24h	q24-48h	Hemo: None CAPD: None CAVH: Dose for GFR 10-50

Urinary retention. Vd decreased in ESRD.

Flecainide	25	12.0-19.5/19-26	52	8.4-9.5	100 mg q12h to 350-400 mg prn	D	100%	100%	50-75%	Hemo: None CAPD: None CAVH: Dose for GFR 10-50

Excretion enhanced in acid urine.

Lidocaine	10	2.0-2.2/1.3-3.0	60-66	1.3-2.2	50 mg over 2 min repeat q 5 min × 3 then 1-4 mg/min	D	100%	100%	100%	Hemo: None CAPD: None CAVH: Dose for GFR 10-50

For definitions of the abbreviations used in the tables, see page 16.

31

Antihypertensive and Cardiovascular Agents (Continued)

Drug, Toxicity Notes	Percent Excreted Unchanged	Half-Life (Normal/ESRD)	Volume of Distribution	Plasma Protein Binding	Dose for Normal Renal Function	Method	Adjustment for Renal Failure GFR, mL/min			Supplement for Dialysis
							>50	10-50	<10	
	%	h	L/kg	%						
Cardiovascular Agents (Continued)										
Antiarrhythmic Agents (Continued)										
Mexiletine Increased renal excretion in acid urine.	10	8-13/16	5.5-6.6	70-75	100-300 mg q6-12h	D	100%	100%	50-75%	Hemo: None CAPD: None CAVH: None
Moricizine	< 1	2/3	> 5.0	95	200-300 q8h	D	100%	100%	100%	Hemo: None CAPD: None CAVH: Dose for GFR 10-50
N-Acetyl-procainamide Hemofiltration useful in poisoning.	80	6-8/42-70	1.5-1.7	10-20	500 mg q6-8h	D,I	100% q6-8h	50% q8-12h	25% q12-18h	Hemo: None CAPD: None CAVH: Dose for GFR 10-50
Procainamide Half-life is acetylator phenotype dependent. Active metabolite is N-acetyl-procainamide. Lupus-like syndrome. Hemofiltration useful in poisoning.	50-60	2.5-4.9/5.3-5.9	2.2	15	350-400 mg q3-4h	I	q4h	q6-12h	q8-24h	Hemo: 200 mg CAPD: None CAVH: Dose for GFR 10-50
Propafenone Half-life is acetylator phenotype dependent.	< 1	5/No data	3.0	> 95	150-300 mg q8h	D	100%	100%	100%	Hemo: None CAPD: None CAVH: Dose for GFR 10-50
Quinidine Increased plasma levels of digoxin and digitoxin in ESRD. Excretion enhanced in acid urine. Hemodialysis useful in poisoning.	20	6/4-14	2.0-3.5	70-95	200-400 mg q4-6h	D	100%	100%	75%	Hemo: 100-200 mg CAPD: None CAVH: Dose for GFR 10-50

Drug				Dose		>50	10-50	<10	Supplement
Tocainide	40	14/22-27	10-20	3.2	200-400 mg q4-6h	D	100%	100%	50%	Hemo: 200 mg CAPD: None CAVH: Dose for GFR 10-50

Excretion decreased in alkaline urine.

Calcium-Channel Blockers

Headache, edema, flushing, dizziness.

Drug				Dose		>50	10-50	<10	Supplement
Amlodipine	<10	35-50/50	>95	21	5.0 mg q24h	D	100%	100%	100%	Hemo: None CAPD: None CAVH: Dose for GFR 10-50

May increase digoxin and cyclosporine levels.

Bepridil	<1	24-48/24-48	No data	No data	No data	D	No data	No data	No data	Hemo: None CAPD: None CAVH: No data

Weak vasodilator and antihypertensive.

Diltiazem	<10	2-8/3.5	98	9-10	10 mg q24h	D	100%	100%	100%	Hemo: None CAPD: None CAVH: Dose for GFR 10-50

Acute renal dysfunction. May exacerbate hyperkalemia. May increase digoxin and cyclosporine levels.

Felodipine	<1	10-14/21-24	99	9-10	10 mg q24h	D	100%	100%	100%	Hemo: None CAPD: None CAVH: Dose for GFR 10-50

May increase digoxin levels.

Isradipine	<5	1.9-4.8/10-11	97	3-4	5-10 mg q24h	D	100%	100%	100%	Hemo: None CAPD: None CAVH: Dose for GFR 10-50

May increase digoxin levels.

Nicardipine	<1	5/5-7	98-99	0.8	20-30 mg tid	D	100%	100%	100%	Hemo: None CAPD: None CAVH: Dose for GFR 10-50

Uremia inhibits hepatic metabolism. May increase digoxin levels.

Nifedipine	<10	4.0-5.5/5-7	97	1.4	10-20 mg q6-8h	D	100%	100%	100%	Hemo: None CAPD: None CAVH: Dose for GFR 10-50

Acute renal dysfunction. Protein binding decreased in ESRD. May increase digoxin levels.

For definitions of the abbreviations used in the tables, see page 16.

Antihypertensive and Cardiovascular Agents (Continued)

Drug, Toxicity Notes	Percent Excreted Unchanged	Plasma Protein Binding	Half-Life (Normal/ ESRD)	Volume of Distribution	Dose for Normal Renal Function	Adjustment for Renal Failure Method	Adjustment for Renal Failure GFR, mL/min >50	Adjustment for Renal Failure GFR, mL/min 10-50	Adjustment for Renal Failure GFR, mL/min <10	Supplement for Dialysis
	%	%	h	L/kg						
Cardiovascular Agents (Continued)										
Calcium-Channel Blockers (Continued)										
Nimodipine May lower blood pressure.	<10	98	1.0-2.8/22	0.9-2.3	30 mg q8h	D	100%	100%	100%	Hemo: None CAPD: None CAVH: Dose for GFR 10-50
Nisoldipine May increase digoxin levels.	<10	99	6.6-7.9/6.8-9.7	2.3-7.1	10 mg bid	D	100%	100%	100%	Hemo: None CAPD: None CAVH: Dose for GFR 10-50
Verapamil Acute renal dysfunction. Active metabolites accumulate particularly with sustained-release forms. May increase digoxin and cyclosporine levels.	<10	83-93	3-7/2.4-4.0	3-6	80 mg q8h	D	100%	100%	100%	Hemo: None CAPD: None CAVH: Dose for GFR 10-50

Cardiac Glycosides

Add to uremic gastrointestinal symptoms. Toxicity enhanced by hypokalemia and hypomagnesemia during dialysis.

Drug, Toxicity Notes	Percent Excreted Unchanged	Plasma Protein Binding	Half-Life (Normal/ ESRD)	Volume of Distribution	Dose for Normal Renal Function	Adjustment for Renal Failure Method	Adjustment for Renal Failure GFR >50	Adjustment for Renal Failure GFR 10-50	Adjustment for Renal Failure GFR <10	Supplement for Dialysis
Digitoxin Increased conversion to digoxin in ESRD (8-10% conversion in normals). Vd decreased by uremia.	20-25	94	144-200/210	0.6	0.1-0.2 mg q24h	D	100%	100%	50-75%	Hemo: None CAPD: None CAVH: Dose for GFR 10-50
Digoxin	76-85	20-30	36-44/80-120	5-8	1.0-1.5 mg load then 0.25-0.5 mg q24h	D,I	100% q24h	25-75% q36h	10-25% q48h	Hemo: None CAPD: None CAVH: Dose for GFR 10-50

Decrease loading dose by 50% in ESRD. Radioimmunoassay may overestimate serum levels in uremia. Clearance decreased by amiodarone, spironolactone, quinidine, verapamil. Hypokalemia, hypomagnesemia enhance toxicity. Vd and total body clearance decreased in ESRD. Serum level 12 hours after dose is best guide in ESRD. Digoxin immune antibodies can treat severe toxicity in ESRD.

Drug	% Excreted	Half-life (Normal/ESRD)	Protein Binding (%)	Vd	Dose for Normal Renal Function	Method	GFR >50	GFR 10–50	GFR <10	Adjustment for Dialysis
Ouabain	40-50	21/60-70	40	No data	0.25 mg load then 0.1 mg q12h	I	q12-24h	q24-36h	q36-48h	Hemo: None CAPD: None CAVH: Dose for GFR 10-50

Diuretics

Natriuretic drugs may cause extracellular fluid volume depletion.

Drug	% Excreted	Half-life (Normal/ESRD)	Protein Binding (%)	Vd	Dose for Normal Renal Function	Method	GFR >50	GFR 10–50	GFR <10	Adjustment for Dialysis
Acetazolamide	100	1.7-5.8/No data	70-90	0.2	250 mg q6-12h	I	q6h	q12h	Avoid	Hemo: No data CAPD: No data CAVH: Avoid
Amiloride	50	6-8/10-144	30-40	5.0-5.2	5.0 mg q24h	D	100%	50%	Avoid	Hemo: Not applicable CAPD: Not applicable CAVH: Not applicable
Bumetanide	33	1.2-1.5/1.5	96	0.2-0.5	1-2 mg q8-12h	D	100%	100%	100%	Hemo: None CAPD: None CAVH: Not applicable
Chlorthalidone	50	44-80/Unknown	76-90	3.9	25 mg q24h	I	q24h	q24h	Avoid	Hemo: Not applicable CAPD: Not applicable CAVH: Not applicable
Ethacrynic acid	20	2-4/No data	90	0.1	50-100 mg tid	I	q8-12h	q8-12h	Avoid	Hemo: None CAPD: None CAVH: Not applicable
Furosemide	67	0.5-1.1/2-4	95	0.07-0.2	40-80 mg bid	D	100%	100%	100%	Hemo: None CAPD: None CAVH: Not applicable
Indapamide	<5	14-18/Unchanged	76-79	0.3-1.3	2.5 mg q24h	D	100%	100%	Avoid	Hemo: None CAPD: None CAVH: Not applicable

Acetazolamide: May potentiate acidosis. Ineffective as diuretic in ESRD. May cause neurologic side effects in dialysis patients.

Amiloride: Hyperkalemia with GFR < 30 mL/min, especially in diabetics. Hyperchloremic metabolic acidosis.

Bumetanide: Ototoxicity increased in ESRD in combination with aminoglycosides. High doses effective in ESRD. Muscle pain, gynecomastia.

Chlorthalidone: Ineffective with low GFR.

Ethacrynic acid: Ototoxicity increased in ESRD in combination with aminoglycosides.

Furosemide: Ototoxicity increased in ESRD, especially in combination with aminoglycosides. High doses effective in ESRD.

Indapamide: Ineffective in ESRD.

For definitions of the abbreviations used in the tables, see page 16.

Antihypertensive and Cardiovascular Agents (Continued)

Drug, Toxicity Notes	Percent Excreted Unchanged	Half-Life (Normal/ ESRD)	Plasma Protein Binding	Volume of Distribution	Dose for Normal Renal Function	Adjustment for Renal Failure Method	>50	10-50	<10	Supplement for Dialysis
	%	h	%	L/kg				GFR, mL/min		

Diuretics (Continued)

Drug, Toxicity Notes	Percent Excreted Unchanged	Half-Life (Normal/ ESRD)	Plasma Protein Binding	Volume of Distribution	Dose for Normal Renal Function	Method	>50	10-50	<10	Supplement for Dialysis
Metolazone	70	4-20/No data	95	1.6	5-10 mg q24h	D	100%	100%	100%	Hemo: None CAPD: None CAVH: Not applicable
High doses effective in ESRD. Gynecomastia, impotence.										
Piretanide	40-60	1.4/1.6-3.4	94	0.3	6-12 mg q24h	D	100%	100%	100%	Hemo: None CAPD: None CAVH: Not applicable
High doses effective in ESRD. Ototoxicity.										
Spironolactone	20-30	10-35/Unchanged	98	No data	25 mg tid-qid	I	q6-12h	q12-24h	Avoid	Hemo: Not applicable CAPD: Not applicable CAVH: Avoid
Active metabolites with long half-life. Hyperkalemia common when GFR < 30, especially in diabetics. Gynecomastia, hyperchloremic acidosis. Increases serum by immunoassay interference.										
Thiazides	> 95	6-8/12-20	40	3.0	25-50 mg bid	D	100%	100%	Avoid	Hemo: Not applicable CAPD: Not applicable CAVH: Not applicable
Usually ineffective with GFR < 30 mL/min. Effective at low GFR in combination with loop diuretic. Hyperuricemia.										
Torasemide	25	2-4/4-5	97-99	0.14-0.19	5.0 mg bid	D	100%	100%	100%	Hemo: None CAPD: None CAVH: Not applicable
High doses effective in ESRD. Ototoxicity.										
Triamterene	5-10	2-12/10	40-70	2.2-3.7	25-50 mg bid	I	q12h	q12h	Avoid	Hemo: Avoid CAPD: Avoid CAVH: Avoid
Hyperkalemia common when GFR < 30, especially in diabetics. Active metabolite with long half-life in ESRD. Folic acid antagonist. Urolithiasis. Crystalluria in acid urine. May cause acute renal failure.										

Cardiovascular Agents (Continued)

Miscellaneous Cardiac Drugs

Amrinone Thrombocytopenia. Nausea, vomiting in ESRD.	10-40	2.6-8.3/No data	20-40	1.3-1.6	5-10 µg/kg/min daily dose <10 mg/kg	D	100%	100%	50-75%	Hemo: No data CAPD: No data CAVH: Dose for GFR 10-50
Dobutamine	<10	2 min/No data	No data	0.25	2.5-15 µg/kg/min	D	100%	100%	100%	Hemo: No data CAPD: No data CAVH: Dose for GFR 10-50
Midodrine Increased blood pressure.	75-80	0.5/No data	No data	No data	No data		5-10 mg q8h	5-10 mg q8h	No data	Hemo: 5 mg q8h CAPD: No data CAVH: Dose for GFR 10-50
Milrinone	80-85	1/1.5-3.0	No data	0.25-0.35	15-75 µg/kg IV load then 2.5-15 mg q6h po	D	100%	100%	50-75%	Hemo: No data CAPD: No data CAVH: Dose for GFR 10-50

Nitrates

Isosorbide Active metabolites with long half-life in ESRD.	10-20	0.15-0.5/4	72	1.5-4.0	10-20 mg tid	D	100%	100%	100%	Hemo: 10-20 mg CAPD: None CAVH: Dose for GFR 10-50
Nitroglycerine	<1	2-4 min/Unchanged	No data	2-3	Many routes & methods	D	100%	100%	100%	Hemo: No data CAPD: No data CAVH: Dose for GFR 10-50

For definitions of the abbreviations used in the tables, see page 16.

Antimicrobial Agents

Dose reduction that results in ineffectively low plasma concentrations is the greatest danger in prescribing antimicrobial agents for patients with renal impairment. Although some antimicrobial agents have a narrow therapeutic index, many are relatively nontoxic. These drugs have a great difference between therapeutic and toxic plasma concentrations. The aminoglycoside antibiotics have a narrow therapeutic range. They are eliminated almost exclusively by glomerular filtration, and accumulation may cause nephrotoxicity and ototoxicity. Patients on aminoglycoside therapy require precise dose reduction, drug-level monitoring, and careful repeated measurements of renal function.

Antimicrobial therapy in patients with renal disease begins with an attempt to isolate the causative organism. Uremic patients with serious infections may not have elevated temperatures. Uremic symptoms or the effects of dialysis may mask nonspecific symptoms of infection. Because patients with renal insufficiency are more likely to have adverse effects from antimicrobial therapy than are patients with normal renal function, culture documentation of bacterial infection is essential. When patients are seriously ill, choose antimicrobial therapy empirically but only after exhaustive attempts to isolate specific pathogens.

The choice of antimicrobial agents includes consideration of potential toxicity. Consider the consequences of inadvertent drug or metabolite accumulation. Side effects, which are rarely seen in patients with normal renal function, occur more frequently in patients with renal failure. For example, seizures from beta-lactam accumulation are rare in patients with sufficient kidney function to prevent drug accumulation, but they may occur in patients with renal impairment when large doses are given.

Mild nephrotoxicity in patients with renal insufficiency may result in overt uremia. A decrease in renal function of as much as 50% from aminoglycoside nephrotoxicity may go unnoticed in patients with normal kidney function. A similar change in patients with creatinine clearances less than 20 mL/min might precipitate the need for dialysis.

Consider the accumulation of metabolic waste products in patients with impaired excretory capacity. The antianabolic effects of tetracycline may cause an increase in the blood urea nitrogen. Avoid drugs that increase metabolic load.

The kidneys eliminate many antimicrobial agents. For most of these drugs, detailed kinetic studies in patients with renal impairment have led to detailed dosing guidelines; however, the derived suggestions are appropriate for the "average" patient and are only a starting point for individualization of therapy.

To reach therapeutic plasma drug levels rapidly, the initial dose of antimicrobial agents for patients with impaired renal function should be the same as that for patients with normal renal function. If substantial edema or ascites is present, a larger initial dose may be necessary. Conversely, dehydrated or severely debilitated patients may require smaller initial doses.

No controlled clinical trials have compared the relative efficacy of modifying drug dose in renal insufficiency by decreasing the individual doses or by increasing the dose interval. When subsequent doses need to be decreased because of diminished renal function, the dose for most antimicrobial agents should be modified by prolonging the dose interval. Because the wide therapeutic range of most of these drugs allows higher peak levels without toxicity and lower trough levels without loss of efficacy, the dose interval often may be extended to 24 hours or more. Extension of the dose interval is more convenient and less expensive; when the clinical situation permits, outpatient parenteral antimicrobial therapy may be given.

To eliminate the risk of ineffectively low drug concentrations in seriously ill patients, the dose interval should not be extended beyond 24 hours. In such patients, a decrease in the individual doses combined with prolonging the dose interval maintains safe, therapeutic drug levels. This combined approach results in therapeutic efficacy, convenience, and cost savings.

Because there is often a direct relation between plasma levels and antimicrobial efficacy or toxicity, drug levels should be measured. Generally, three or four doses should be given before levels are measured to ensure that steady-state concentrations have been established. For some drugs, both maximum and minimum concentrations are relevant. Peak levels are most meaningful when measured after rapid drug distribution has occurred. Minimum plasma drug concentrations should be measured immediately before the next dose is to be given. These trough levels are measures of elimination and reflect more closely the potential drug accumulation in patients with renal failure. Drug level monitoring is particularly important in patients with unstable renal function.

Antimicrobial Agents

Drug, Toxicity Notes	Percent Excreted Unchanged	Plasma Protein Binding	Volume of Distribution	Half-Life (Normal/ ESRD)	Dose for Normal Renal Function	Method	Adjustment for Renal Failure GFR, mL/min			Supplement for Dialysis
							>50	10-50	<10	
	%	%	L/kg	h						
Antibacterial Antibiotics										

Aminoglycoside Antibiotics

Nephrotoxic. Ototoxic. Toxicity worse when hyperbilirubinemic. Measure serum levels for efficacy and toxicity. Peritoneal absorption increases with presence of inflammation. Vd increases with edema, obesity, and ascites.

Drug, Toxicity Notes	Percent Excreted Unchanged	Plasma Protein Binding	Volume of Distribution	Half-Life (Normal/ ESRD)	Dose for Normal Renal Function	Method	>50	10-50	<10	Supplement for Dialysis
Amikacin Monitor levels.	95	< 5	0.22-0.29	1.4-2.3/17-150	7.5 mg/kg q12h	D,I	60-90% q12h or 100% q12-24h	30-70% q12-18h or 100% q24-48h	20-30% q24-48h q48-72h	Hemo: 1/2 full dose after dialysis CAPD: 15-20 mg/L/d CAVH: Dose for GFR 10-50 & measure levels
Gentamicin Concurrent penicillins may result in subtherapeutic aminoglycoside levels.	95	< 5	0.23-0.26	1.8/20-60	1.7 mg/kg q8h	D,I	60-90% q8-12h or 100% q12-24h	30-70% q12h or 100% q24-48h	20-30% q24-48h q48-72h	Hemo: 1/2 full dose after dialysis CAPD: 3-4 mg/L/d CAVH: Dose for GFR 10-50 & measure levels
Kanamycin	50-90	< 5	0.19-0.23	1.8-5.0/40-96	7.5 mg/kg q12h	D,I	60-90% q12h or 100% q12-24h	30-70% q12-18h or 100% q24-48h	20-30% q24-48h q48-72h	Hemo: 1/2 full dose after dialysis CAPD: 15-20 mg/L/d CAVH: Dose for GFR 10-50 & measure levels

Drug					Dose	D/I	GFR >50	GFR 10-50	GFR <10	Dialysis
Netilmicin	95	1-3/35-72	<5	0.16-0.30	2 mg/kg q8h	D,I	50-90% q8-12h or 100% q12-24h	20-60% q12h or 100% q24-48h	10-20% q24-48h or 100% q48-72h	Hemo: 1/2 full dose after dialysis CAPD: 3-4 mg/L/d CAVH: Dose for GFR 10-50 & measure levels
May be less ototoxic than other members of class.										
Streptomycin	70	2.5/100	35	0.26	7.5 mg/kg q12h (1.0 g q24h for tuberculosis)	I	q24h	q24-72h	q72-96h	Hemo: 1/2 normal dose after dialysis CAPD: 20-40 mg/L/d CAVH: Dose for GFR 10-50 & measure levels
May be less nephrotoxic than other members of class.										
Tobramycin	95	2.5/27-60	<5	0.22-0.33	1.7 mg/kg q8h	D,I	60-90% q8-12h or 100% q12-24h	30-70% q12h or 100% q24-48h	20-30% q24-48h or 100% q48-72	Hemo: 1/2 full dose after dialysis CAPD: 3-4 mg/L/d CAVH: Dose for GFR 10-50 & measure levels
Concurrent penicillins may result in subtherapeutic aminoglycoside levels.										

Cephalosporin Antibiotics

Rare allergic interstitial nephritis. Absorbed well when given intraperitoneally. May cause bleeding from impaired prothrombin biosynthesis.

Drug					Dose	D/I	GFR >50	GFR 10-50	GFR <10	Dialysis
Cefaclor	70	1/3	25	0.24-0.35	250-500 mg tid	D	100%	50-100%	50%	Hemo: 250 mg after dialysis CAPD: 250 mg q8-12h CAVH: Not applicable
Cefadroxil	70-90	1.4/22	20	0.31	0.5-1.0 g q12h	I	q12h	q12-24h	q24-48h	Hemo: 0.5-1.0 g after dialysis CAPD: 0.5 g/d CAVH: Not applicable
Cefamandole	50-100	1/6-11	75	0.16-0.25	0.5-1.0 g q4-8h	I	q6h	q6-8h	q12h	Hemo: 0.5-1.0 g after dialysis CAPD: 0.5-1.0 g q12h CAVH: Dose for GFR 10-50

For definitions of the abbreviations used in the tables, see page 16.

Antimicrobial Agents (Continued)

Drug, Toxicity Notes	Percent Excreted Unchanged	Half-Life (Normal/ESRD)	Plasma Protein Binding	Volume of Distribution	Dose for Normal Renal Function	Adjustment for Renal Failure Method	GFR, mL/min >50	10-50	<10	Supplement for Dialysis
	%	h	%	L/kg						
Antibacterial Antibiotics (Continued)										
Cephalosporin Antibiotics (Continued)										
Cefazolin	75-95	2/40-70	80	0.13-0.22	0.5-1.5 g q6h	I	q8h	q12h	q24-48h	Hemo: 0.5-1.0 g after dialysis CAPD: 0.5 g q12h CAVH: Dose for GFR 10-50
Cefepime	85	2.2/18	16	0.3	250-2000 mg q8h	I	q12h	q16-24h	q24-48h	Hemo: 1.0 g after dialysis CAPD: Dose for GFR <10 CAVH: Not recommended
Cefixime 400 mg/d to treat peritonitis.	18-50	3.1/12	50	0.6-0.11	200 mg q12h	D	100%	75%	50%	Hemo: 300 mg after dialysis CAPD: 200 mg/d CAVH: Not recommended
Cefmenoxime	70	0.8-1.3/6-12	43-75	0.27-0.37	1.0 g q6h	D,I	1.0 g q8h	0.75 g q8h	0.75 g q12h	Hemo: 0.75 g after dialysis CAPD: 0.75 g q12h CAVH: Dose for GFR 10-50
Cefmetazole Probenecid doubles half-life.	85	1.2/21	75	0.18	2.0 g q6-12h	I	q16h	q24h	q48h	Hemo: Dose after dialysis CAPD: Dose for GFR <10 CAVH: Dose for GFR 10-50
Cefonicid	95	4/17-59	96	0.09-0.18	1.0 g q24h	D,I	0.5 g q24h	0.1-0.5g q24h	0.1 g q24h	Hemo: None CAPD: None CAVH: None

Drug	%	t½ norm/ESRD	%	Vd	Normal dose	Method	GFR >50	GFR 10-50	GFR <10	Supplement
Cefoperazone	20	1.6-2.5/2.9	90	0.14-0.20	1-2 g q12h	D	100%	100%	100%	Hemo: 1.0 g after dialysis CAPD: None CAVH: None

Displaced from protein by bilirubin. Reduce dose by 50% for jaundice. May prolong prothrombin time.

Drug	%	t½ norm/ESRD	%	Vd	Normal dose	Method	GFR >50	GFR 10-50	GFR <10	Supplement
Ceforanide	85	3/25	80	0.17	0.5-1.0 g q12h	I	q12h	q12-24h	q24-48h	Hemo: 0.5-1.0 g after dialysis CAPD: None CAVH: 1.0 g/d
Cefotaxime	60	1/15	37	0.15-0.55	1.0 g q6h	I	q6h	q8-12h	q24h	Hemo: 1.0 g after dialysis CAPD: 1.0 g/d CAVH: 1.0 g q12h

Active metabolite in ESRD. Reduce dose further for combined hepatic and renal failure.

Drug	%	t½ norm/ESRD	%	Vd	Normal dose	Method	GFR >50	GFR 10-50	GFR <10	Supplement
Cefotetan	75	3.5/13-25	85	0.15	1-2 g q12h	D	100%	50%	25%	Hemo: 1.0 g after dialysis CAPD: 1.0 g/d CAVH: 750 mg q12h
Cefoxitin	80	1/13-23	41-75	0.2	1-2 g q6-8h	I	q8h	q8-12h	q24-48h	Hemo: 1.0 g after dialysis CAPD: 1.0 g/d CAVH: Dose for GFR 10-50

May produce false increase in serum creatinine by interference with assay.

Drug	%	t½ norm/ESRD	%	Vd	Normal dose	Method	GFR >50	GFR 10-50	GFR <10	Supplement
Cefpodoxime	30	2.5/26	26	0.6-1.2	200 mg q12h	I	q12h	q16h	q24-48h	Hemo: 200 mg after dialysis only CAPD: Dose for GFR <10 CAVH: Not applicable
Cefprozil	65	1.7/6	40	0.65	500 mg q12h	D,I	250 mg q12h	250 mg q12-16h	250 mg q24h	Hemo: 250 mg after dialysis CAPD: Dose for GFR <10 CAVH: Dose for GFR <10
Ceftazidime	60-85	1.2/13-25	17	0.28-0.4	1-2 g q8h	I	q8-12h	q24-48h	q48h	Hemo: 1.0 g after dialysis CAPD: 0.5 g/d CAVH: Dose for GFR 10-50
Ceftibuten	60-75	1.5-2.7/22	70	0.2	400 mg q24h	D	100%	50%	25%	Hemo: 300 mg after dialysis only CAPD: No data: Dose for GFR < 10 CAVH: Dose for GFR 10-50

For definitions of the abbreviations used in the tables, see page 16.

Antimicrobial Agents (Continued)

Drug, Toxicity Notes	Percent Excreted Unchanged	Half-Life (Normal/ ESRD)	Plasma Protein Binding	Volume of Distribution	Dose for Normal Renal Function	Adjustment for Renal Failure				Supplement for Dialysis
						Method	GFR, mL/min			
							>50	10-50	<10	
	%	h	%	L/kg						

Antibacterial Antibiotics (Continued)

Cephalosporin Antibiotics (Continued)

Drug, Toxicity Notes	Percent Excreted Unchanged	Half-Life (Normal/ ESRD)	Plasma Protein Binding	Volume of Distribution	Dose for Normal Renal Function	Method	>50	10-50	<10	Supplement for Dialysis
Ceftizoxime	57-100	1.4/35	28-50	0.26-0.42	1-2 g q8-12h	I	q8-12h	q12-24h	q24h	Hemo: 1.0 g after dialysis CAPD: 0.5-1.0 g/d CAVH: Dose for GFR 10-50
Ceftriaxone	30-65	7-9/12-24	90	0.12-0.18	0.2-1.0 g q12h	D	100%	100%	100%	Hemo: Dose after dialysis CAPD: 750 mg q12h CAVH: Dose for GFR 10-50
Cefuroxime axetil Malabsorbed in presence of H2 blockers. Absorbed better with food.	90	1.2/17	35-50	0.13-1.8	250-500 mg q12h	D	100%	100%	100%	Hemo: Dose after dialysis CAPD: Dose for GFR <10 CAVH: Not applicable
Cefuroxime sodium	90	1.2/17	33	0.13-1.8	0.75-1.5 g q8h	I	q8h	q8-12h	q12h	Hemo: Dose after dialysis CAPD: Dose for GFR <10 CAVH: 1.0 g q12h
Cephalexin	98	0.7/16	20	0.35	250-500 mg q6h	I	q8h	q12h	q12h	Hemo: Dose after dialysis CAPD: Dose for GFR <10 CAVH: Not applicable
Cephalothin	60-90	0.5-1/3-18	65	0.26	0.5-2.0 g q6h	I	q6h	q6-8h	q12h	Hemo: Dose after dialysis CAPD: 1.0 g q12h CAVH: 1.0 g q8h

Drug				Dose					
Cephapirin	60	0.4/2.5	45-60	0.22	0.5-2.0 g q6h	I	q6h	q6-8h	q12h	Hemo: Dose after dialysis CAPD: 1.0 g q12h CAVH: 1.0 g q8h
Cephradine	100	0.7-1.3/6-15	10	0.25-0.46	0.25-2.0 g q6h	D	100%	50%	25%	Hemo: Dose after dialysis CAPD: Dose for GFR <10 CAVH: Not applicable
Moxalactam	61-79	2.3/18-23	35-59	0.18-0.4	1-2 g q8-12h	I	q8-12h	q12-24h	q24-48h	Hemo: Dose after dialysis CAPD: Dose for GFR <10 CAVH: Dose for GFR 10-50

Sodium, 3.8 mEq/g. Platelet dysfunction at high doses. Monitor prothrombin time or give vitamin K.

Miscellaneous Antibacterial Antibiotics

Drug				Dose					
Azithromycin	6-12	10-60/?	8-50	18	250-500 mg q24h	D	100%	100%	100%	Hemo: None CAPD: None CAVH: None

ESRD dosing recommendations based on extrapolation as no data are yet available.

Drug				Dose					
Aztreonam	75	1.7-2.9/6-8	45-60	0.5-1.0	12.5 mg/kg q8-12h	D	100%	50-75%	25%	Hemo: 0.5 g after dialysis CAPD: Dose for GFR <10 CAVH: Dose for GFR 10-50
Chloramphenicol	10	1.6-3.3/3-7	45-60	0.5-1.0	12.5 mg/kg q6h	D	100%	100%	100%	Hemo: Dose after dialysis CAPD: None CAVH: None
Cilastin	60	1/12	44	0.22	With imipenem	D	100%	50%	Avoid	Hemo: Avoid CAPD: Avoid CAVH: Avoid

Unnecessary in renal failure.

Drug				Dose					
Clarithromycin	15-25	2.3-6.0/?	70	2-4	0.5-1.0 g q12h	D	100%	75%	50-75%	Hemo: No data: Dose after dialysis CAPD: None CAVH: None
Clavulanic acid	40	1/3-4	30	0.3	100 mg q4-6h	D	100%	100%	50-75%	Hemo: Dose after dialysis CAPD: Dose for GFR <10 CAVH: Dose for GFR 10-5

Used only in fixed combination with ticarcillin or amoxicillin.

For definitions of the abbreviations used in the tables, see page 16.

Antimicrobial Agents (Continued)

Drug, Toxicity Notes	Percent Excreted Unchanged	Half-Life (Normal/ ESRD)	Plasma Protein Binding	Volume of Distribution	Dose for Normal Renal Function	Adjustment for Renal Failure				Supplement for Dialysis
						Method	GFR, mL/min			
							>50	10-50	<10	
	%	h	%	L/kg						

Miscellaneous Antibacterial Antibiotics (Continued)

Antibacterial Antibiotics (Continued)

Drug, Toxicity Notes	Percent Excreted Unchanged	Half-Life (Normal/ESRD)	Plasma Protein Binding	Volume of Distribution	Dose for Normal Renal Function	Method	>50	10-50	<10	Supplement for Dialysis
Clindamycin	10	2-4/3-5	60-95	0.6-1.2	150-300 mg q6h	D	100%	100%	100%	Hemo: None CAPD: None CAVH: None
Clofazamine	<1	10-70 d (?)/No data	No data	No data	100-300 mg q24h		No data: 100%	No data: 100%	No data: 100%	Hemo: No data: None CAPD: No data: None CAVH: No data
Dapsone Hemolytic anemia with G6PD deficiency.	5-20	20-30/No data	70-90	1.0-1.5	50-100 mg q24h for malaria prophylaxis once weekly		No data: 100%	No data	No data	Hemo: No data: None CAPD: No data: Dose for GFR < 10 CAVH: No data
Dirithromycin Nonenzymatically hydrolyzed to active compound erythromycylamine.	1-3	30-44/No data	15-30	>10	500 mg q24h		100%	100%	100%	Hemo: None CAPD: No data: None CAVH: Dose for GFR 10-50
Erythromycin Ototoxicity with high doses in ESRD. Vd increases in ESRD.	15	1.4/5-6	60-95	0.6-1.2	150-300 mg q6h	D	100%	100%	50-75%	Hemo: None CAPD: None CAVH: None
Imipenem Seizures in ESRD. Nonrenal clearance in acute renal failure is less than in chronic renal failure. Administered with cilastin to prevent nephrotoxicity of renal metabolite.	20-70	1/4	13-21	0.17-0.3	0.25-1.0 g q6h	D	100%	50%	25%	Hemo: Dose after dialysis CAPD: Dose for GFR <10 CAVH: Dose for GFR 10-50

Drug				Dose					
Lincomycin	10-15	4-5/10-20	70-80	0.31-0.6	0.5 g q6h	I	q6h	q6-12h	q12-24h	Hemo: None CAPD: None CAVH: Not applicable
Loracarbef	85-95	0.8-1.3/32	25	0.3-0.4	200-400 12h	I	q12h	q24h	q3-5d	Hemo: Dose after dialysis CAPD: No data: Dose for GFR <10 CAVH: Dose for GFR 10-50
Meropenem	65	1.1/6-8	Low	0.35	500-1000 mg q6h	D,I	500 mg q6h	250-500 mg q12h	250-500 mg q24h	Hemo: Dose after dialysis CAPD: Dose for GFR <10 CAVH: Dose for GFR 10-50
Methenamine mandelate	High	4/No data	No data	No data	1.0 g q6h	D	100%	Avoid	Avoid	Hemo: Not applicable CAPD: Not applicable CAVH: Not applicable
Metronidazole	20	6-14/7-21	20	0.25-0.85	7.5 mg/kg q6h	D	100%	100%	50% *(handwritten: 50% 500.28 upo)*	Hemo: Dose after dialysis CAPD: Dose for GFR <10 CAVH: Dose for GFR 10-50
Metronidazole — *Metabolites accumulate. Rare drug-induced lupus.*									
Nitrofurantoin	30-40	0.5/1	20-60	0.3-0.7	50-100 mg q6h	D	100%	Avoid	Avoid	Hemo: Not applicable CAPD: Not applicable CAVH: Not applicable
Spectinomycin	35-90	1.6/16-29	5-20	0.25	2-4 g once	D	100%	100%	100%	Hemo: None CAPD: None CAVH: None
Sulbactam	50-80	1/10-21	30	0.25-0.5	0.75-1.5 q6-8h	I	q6-8h	q12-24h	q24-48h	Hemo: Dose after dialysis CAPD: 0.75-1.5 g/d CAVH: 750 mg q12h
Sulbactam — *Beta-lactamase inhibitor combined with ampicillin.*									
Sulfamethoxazole	70	10/20-50	50	0.28-0.38	1.0 g q8h	I	q12h	q18h	q24h	Hemo: 1.0 g after dialysis CAPD: 1.0 g/d CAVH: Dose for GFR 10-50
Sulfamethoxazole — *Recommendation if given as single agent. Protein binding decreased in ESRD. Use normal dosing for urinary tract infection in ESRD.*									

For definitions of the abbreviations used in the tables, see page 16.

Antimicrobial Agents (Continued)

Drug, Toxicity Notes	Percent Excreted Unchanged %	Half-Life (Normal/ESRD) h	Plasma Protein Binding %	Volume of Distribution L/kg	Dose for Normal Renal Function	Adjustment for Renal Failure Method	GFR, mL/min >50	10-50	<10	Supplement for Dialysis
Miscellaneous Antibacterial Antibiotics (Continued)										
Sulfisoxazole	70	3-7/6-12	85	0.14-0.28	1-2 g q6h	I	q6h	q8-12h	q12-24h	Hemo: 2.0 g after dialysis CAPD: 3.0 g/d CAVH: Not applicable
Protein binding decreased in ESRD. Use normal dosing for urinary tract infection in ESRD.										
Tazobactam	65	1/7	22	0.21	1.5-2.25 g q24h	D	100%	75%	50%	Hemo: 1/3 dose after dialysis CAPD: Dose for GFR <10 CAVH: Dose for GFR 10-50
Combined with piperacillin; dose adjustments determined by piperacillin.										
Teicoplanin	40-60	33-190/62-230	60-90	0.5-1.2	6.0 mg/kg q24h	I	q24h	q48h	q72h	Hemo: Dose for GFR <10 CAPD: Dose for GFR <10 CAVH: Dose for GFR 10-50
Trimethoprim	40-70	9-13/20-49	30-70	1.0-2.2	100-200 mg q12h	I	q12h	q18h	q24h	Hemo: Dose after dialysis CAPD: q24h CAVH: q18h
Can cause hyperkalemia.										
Vancomycin	90-100	6-8/200-250	10-50	0.47-1.1	500 mg q6h or 1 g q12h	D,I	1.0 gm q12-24h	1.0 gm q24-96h	1.0 gm q4-7d	Hemo: Dose for GFR <10 CAPD: Dose for GFR <10 CAVH: Dose for GFR 10-50
In patients with renal failure, vancomycin serum concentrations may be overestimated by fluorescence polarization immunoassay (FPIA) and radioimmunoassay (RIA) testing methods due to interference from the biologically inactive vancomycin breakdown product (crystalline degradation product [CDP-1]). The monoclonal-enzyme multiplied immunotechnique (EMIT) method is not affected by CDP-1 accumulation.										

Penicillins

Drug				Dose	Method	>50	10-50	<10	Supplement
Amoxicillin	50-70	0.9-2.3/5-20	15-25	0.26	250-500 mg q8h	I	q8h	q8-12h	q24h	Hemo: Dose after dialysis CAPD: 250 mg q12h CAVH: Not applicable
Ampicillin	30-90	0.8-1.5/7-20	20	0.17-0.31	250 mg-2g q6h	I	q6h	q6-12h	q12-24h	Hemo: Dose after dialysis CAPD: 250 mg q12h CAVH: Dose for GFR 10-50
Azlocillin	50-75	0.8-1.5/5-6	30	0.18-0.27	2-3 g q4h	I	q4-6h	q6-8h	q8h	Hemo: Dose after dialysis CAPD: Dose for GFR <10 CAVH: Dose for GFR 10-50

Sodium, 2.7 mEq/g. May cause hypokalemic metabolic alkalosis.

Drug				Dose	Method	>50	10-50	<10	Supplement
Dicloxacillin	35-70	0.7/1-2	95	0.16	250-500 mg q6h	D	100%	100%	100%	Hemo: None CAPD: None CAVH: Not applicable
Methicillin	25-80	0.5-1/4	35-60	0.31	1-2 g q4h	I	q4-6h	q6-8h	q8-12h	Hemo: None CAPD: None CAVH: Dose for GFR 10-50
Mezlocillin	65	0.6-1.2/2.6-5.4	20-46	0.18	1.5-4.0 g q4-6h	I	q4-6h	q6-8h	q8h	Hemo: None CAPD: None CAVH: Dose for GFR 10-50

Schedule next dose after dialysis. Reduce dose further for combined liver and kidney disease.

Drug				Dose	Method	>50	10-50	<10	Supplement
Nafcillin	35	0.5/1.2	85	0.35	1-2 g q4-6h	D	100%	100%	100%	Hemo: None CAPD: None CAVH: Dose for GFR 10-50
Penicillin G	60-85	0.5/6-20	50	0.3-0.42	0.5-4 million U q6h	D	100%	75%	20-50%	Hemo: Dose after dialysis CAPD: Dose for GFR <10 CAVH: Dose for GFR 10-50

Seizures. False-positive urine protein reactions. Six million units/d upper limit dose in ESRD.

Drug				Dose	Method	>50	10-50	<10	Supplement
Penicillin VK	60-90	0.6/4.1	50-80	0.5	250 mg q6h	D	100%	100%	100%	Hemo: Dose after dialysis CAPD: Dose for GFR <10 CAVH: Not applicable

For definitions of the abbreviations used in the tables, see page 16.

51

Antimicrobial Agents (Continued)

Drug, Toxicity Notes	Percent Excreted Unchanged	Half-Life (Normal/ESRD)	Plasma Protein Binding	Volume of Distribution	Dose for Normal Renal Function	Adjustment for Renal Failure				Supplement for Dialysis
						Method	GFR, mL/min			
							>50	10-50	<10	
	%	h	%	L/kg						
Antibacterial Antibiotics (Continued)										
Penicillins (Continued)										
Piperacillin, Sodium, 1.9 mEq/g.	75-90	0.8-1.5/3.3-5.1	30	0.18-0.30	3-4 g q4h	I	q4-6h	q6-8h	q8h	Hemo: Dose after dialysis CAPD: Dose for GFR <10 CAVH: Dose for GFR 10-50
Ticarcillin, Sodium, 5.2 mEq/g.	85	1.2/11-16	45-60	0.14-0.21	3.0 g q4h	D,I	1-2 g q4h	1-2 g q8h	1-2 g q12	Hemo: 3.0 g after dialysis CAPD: Dose for GFR <10 CAVH: Dose for GFR 10-50

Quinolone Antibiotics

Most agents in this group are malabsorbed in the presence of compounds that contain metals such as magnesium, calcium, aluminum, and iron. Theophylline metabolism is impaired by some members of this group. Higher oral doses may be needed to treat CAPD peritonitis.

Drug, Toxicity Notes	Percent Excreted Unchanged	Half-Life (Normal/ESRD)	Plasma Protein Binding	Volume of Distribution	Dose for Normal Renal Function	Adjustment for Renal Failure				Supplement for Dialysis
	%	h	%	L/kg		Method	>50	10-50	<10	
Cinoxacin	55	1.2/12	63	0.25	500 mg q12h	D	100%	50%	Avoid	Hemo: Avoid CAPD: Avoid CAVH: Avoid
Ciprofloxacin	50-70	3-6/6-9	20-40	2.5	500-750 mg (400 mg if intravenous) q12h	D	100%	50-75%	50%	Hemo: 250 mg q12h (200 mg if iv) CAPD: 250 mg q8h (200 mg if iv) CAVH: 200 mg iv q12h

Poorly absorbed with antacids, sucralfate, and phosphate binders. Intravenous dose 1/3 of oral dose. Decreases phenytoin levels.

Drug										
Fleroxacin	70	9-13/21-28	20	1.1-2.4	400 mg q12h	D	100%	50-75%	50%	Hemo: Dose for GFR <10 CAPD: 400 mg/d CAVH: Not applicable
Levofloxacin L-isomer of ofloxacin: appears to have similar pharmacokinetics and toxicities.	67-87	4-8/76	24-38	1.1-1.5	500 mg q24h	D	100%	250 mg q24-48h (500 mg initial dose)	250 mg q48h (500 mg initial dose)	Hemo: Dose for GFR <10 CAPD: Dose for GFR <10 CAVH: Dose for GFR 10-50
Lomefloxacin	76	8/44	15	1.8-3.1	400 mg q24h	D	100%	200-400 mg q48h	50%	Hemo: Dose for GFR <10 CAPD: Dose for GFR <10 CAVH: Not applicable
Nalidixic acid	High	6/21	90	0.25-0.35	1.0 g q6h	D	100%	Avoid	Avoid	Hemo: Avoid CAPD: Avoid CAVH: Not applicable
Norfloxacin	30	3.5-6.5/8	14	< 0.5	400 mg q12h	I	q12h	q12-24h	400 mg q24h	Hemo: Dose for GFR <10 CAPD: Dose for GFR <10 CAVH: Not applicable
Ofloxacin	68-80	5-8/28-37	25	1.5-2.5	200-400 mg q12h	D	100%	200-400 mg q24h	200 mg q24h	Hemo: 100-200 mg after dialysis CAPD: Dose for GFR <10 CAVH: 300 mg/d
Pefloxacin Excellent bidirectional transperitoneal movement.	11	10-12/12-15	25-43	2.0	400 mg q24h	D	100%	100%	100%	Hemo: None CAPD: None CAVH: Dose for GFR 10-50
Sparfloxacin	10	15-20/38.5	35-55	4.5	400 mg q24h	D,I	100%	50-75%	50% q48h	Hemo: No data: Dose for GFR < 10 CAPD: No data CAVH: Dose for GFR 10-50

For definitions of the abbreviations used in the tables, see page 16.

Antimicrobial Agents (Continued)

Drug, Toxicity Notes	Percent Excreted Unchanged	Half-Life (Normal/ESRD)	Plasma Protein Binding	Volume of Distribution	Dose for Normal Renal Function	Method	GFR, mL/min >50	GFR, mL/min 10-50	GFR, mL/min <10	Supplement for Dialysis
	%	h	%	L/kg						

Tetracycline Antibiotics
Potentiate acidosis. Increase BUN, phosphorus. Antianabolic.

Drug, Toxicity Notes	Percent Excreted Unchanged	Half-Life (Normal/ESRD)	Plasma Protein Binding	Volume of Distribution	Dose for Normal Renal Function	Method	GFR, mL/min >50	GFR, mL/min 10-50	GFR, mL/min <10	Supplement for Dialysis
Antibacterial Antibiotics (Continued)										
Doxycycline Group drug of choice for decreased renal function. Not antianabolic.	35-45	15-2 /18-25	80-90	0.75	100 mg q24h	D	100%	100%	100%	Hemo: None CAPD: None CAVH: Dose for GFR 10-5
Minocycline	6-10	12-16/12-18	70	1.0-1.5	100 mg q12h	D	100%	100%	100%	Hemo: None CAPD: None CAVH: Dose for GFR 10-50
Tetracycline Avoid in ESRD.	48-60	6-10/57-108	55-90	> 0.7	250-500 mg qid	I	q8-12h	q12-24h	q24h	Hemo: None CAPD: None CAVH: Dose for GFR 10-5
Antifungal Antibiotics										
Amphotericin B	5-10	24 (up to 15 d)/ Unchanged	90	4.0	20-50 mg q24h	I	q24h	q24h	q24-36h	Hemo: None CAPD: Dose for GFR <10 CAVH: Dose for GFR 10-50

Nephrotoxic. Renal tubular acidosis, potassium wasting. Nephrogenic diabetes insipidus. Ineffective for urinary tract infection in ESRD. Toxicity lessened by saline loading and worsened by concomitant cyclosporin A, aminoglycosides, or pentamidine.

Drug	Percent Excreted Unchanged	Half-life (Normal/ESRD)	Protein Binding	Vd	Dose for Normal Renal Function	Method	GFR >50	GFR 10-50	GFR <10	Adjustment for Dialysis
Amphotericin B colloidal dispersion		24-30/ ? Unchanged	90	4.0	3.0-6.0 mg/kg q24h	I	q24h	q24h	q24-36h	Hemo: None CAPD: Dose for GFR <10 CAVH: Dose for GFR 10-50

Less nephrotoxicity than standard amphotericin B; and Vd appear to be the same as with standard amphotericin B; no data on pharmacokinetics in renal failure.

Drug	Percent Excreted Unchanged	Half-life (Normal/ESRD)	Protein Binding	Vd	Dose for Normal Renal Function	Method	GFR >50	GFR 10-50	GFR <10	Adjustment for Dialysis
Amphotericin B lipid complex	<1	19-45/? Unchanged	90	1.7-3.9	5 mg/kg q24h	I	q24h	q24h	q24-36h	Hemo: None CAPD: Dose for GFR <10 CAVH: Dose for GFR 10-50

There are 630 mg NaCl in a 350 mg dose (9 mg NaCl/mL). Less nephrotoxicity than standard amphotericin B formulation; may have larger Vd and longer $T_{1/2}$ compared with standard amphotericin B preparation; no data on pharmacokinetics in renal failure.

Drug	Percent Excreted Unchanged	Half-life (Normal/ESRD)	Protein Binding	Vd	Dose for Normal Renal Function	Method	GFR >50	GFR 10-50	GFR <10	Adjustment for Dialysis
Fluconazole	70	22/No data	12	0.7	200-400 mg q24h	D	100%	50%	50%	Hemo: 200 mg after dialysis CAPD: Dose for GFR <10 CAVH: Dose for GFR 10-50

Give an initial dose equal to the dose for normal renal function.

Drug	Percent Excreted Unchanged	Half-life (Normal/ESRD)	Protein Binding	Vd	Dose for Normal Renal Function	Method	GFR >50	GFR 10-50	GFR <10	Adjustment for Dialysis
Flucytosine	90	3-6/75-200	<10	0.6	37.5 mg/kg q6h	I	q12h	q16h	q24h	Hemo: Dose after dialysis CAPD: 0.5-1.0 g/d CAVH: Dose for GFR 10-50

Hepatic dysfunction. Marrow suppression more common in azotemic patients.

Drug	Percent Excreted Unchanged	Half-life (Normal/ESRD)	Protein Binding	Vd	Dose for Normal Renal Function	Method	GFR >50	GFR 10-50	GFR <10	Adjustment for Dialysis
Griseofulvin	1	14/20	No data	1.6	125-250 mg q6h	D	100%	100%	100%	Hemo: None CAPD: None CAVH: None
Itraconazole	35	21/25	99	10	100-200 mg q12h	D	100%	100%	50%	Hemo: 100 mg q12-24h CAPD: 100 mg q12-24h CAVH: 100 mg q12-24h
Ketoconazole	13	1.5-3.3/3.3	99	1.9-3.6	200 mg q24h	D	100%	100%	100%	Hemo: None CAPD: None CAVH: None
Miconazole	1	20-24/Unchanged	90	Large	200-1200 mg q8h	D	100%	100%	100%	Hemo: None CAPD: None CAVH: None

For definitions of the abbreviations used in the tables, see page 16.

55

Antimicrobial Agents (Continued)

Drug, Toxicity Notes	Percent Excreted Unchanged	Half-Life (Normal/ESRD)	Plasma Protein Binding	Volume of Distribution	Dose for Normal Renal Function	Adjustment for Renal Failure		GFR, mL/min		Supplement for Dialysis
	%	h	%	L/kg		Method	>50	10-50	<10	
Antimycobacterial Antibiotics										
Capreomycin	50	2	No data	No data	1.0 g q24h	I	q24h	q24h	q48h	Hemo: Give dose after HD only / CAPD: None / CAVH: Dose for GFR 10-50
Nephrotoxic. Potentiates neuromuscular blockade.										
Cycloserine	65	0.5	No data	0.11-0.26	250 mg q12h	I	q12h	q12-24h	q24h	Hemo: None / CAPD: None / CAVH: Dose for GFR 10-50
CNS toxicity.										
Ethambutol	75-90	4/5-15	10-30	1.6-3.2	15-25 mg/kg q24h	I	q24h	q24-36h	q48h	Hemo: Dose after dialysis / CAPD: Dose for GFR <10 / CAVH: Dose for GFR 10-50
Decreases visual acuity. Alternate dose of 25 mg/kg 4-6h before each thrice weekly hemodialysis treatment has been suggested.										
Ethionamide	1	2.1	30	No data	250-500 mg q12h	D	100%	100%	50%	Hemo: None / CAPD: None / CAVH: None
Isoniazid	5-30	0.7-4/1-17	4-30	0.75	300 mg q24h	D	100%	100%	100%	Hemo: Dose after dialysis / CAPD: Dose for GFR <10 / CAVH: Dose for GFR <10
Supplement with 50-100 mg pyridoxine daily to prevent neurotoxicity.										
PAS	80	1.0	15-50	0.11-24	50 mg/kg q8h	D	100%	50-75%	50%	Hemo: Dose after dialysis / CAPD: Dose for GFR <10 / CAVH: Dose for GFR <10
Significant sodium load.										

Drug				Dose		GFR >50	GFR 10–50	GFR <10	Dialysis
Pyrazinimide	1-3	9/26	5	0.75-1.3	25-30 mg/kg q24h (up to 2.5 g)	D	100%	100%	50-100%	Hemo: 40 mg/kg 24h prior each 3x/wk dialysis; CAPD: 100%; CAVH: No data

Impairs urate excretion. Can precipitate gout. Alternate dose of 25-30 mg/kg after each thrice-weekly hemodialysis treatment has been suggested.

Antiparasitic Antibiotics

Drug				Dose		GFR >50	GFR 10–50	GFR <10	Dialysis
Atovaquone	< 1	55-77/No data	99	No data	750 mg q12h (susp)	D	No data: 100%	No data: 100%	No data: 100%	Hemo: No; CAPD: No data: None; CAVH: No data: Dose for GFR 10-50
Chloroquine	40	7-14 d/5-50 d	50-65	> 100	1.5 g over 3 days	D	100%	100%	50%	Hemo: None; CAPD: None; CAVH: None
Mefloquine	< 1	15-33 d/No data	98	20	1250 mg (250 mg weekly for prophylaxis) one-time dose		100%	No data: 100%	No data: 100%	Hemo: None; CAPD: No data: None; CAVH: No data: Dose for GFR 10-50
Pentamidine	< 5	29/73-118	69	3-4	4.0 mg/kg q24h	I	q24h	q24h	q24-36h	Hemo: None; CAPD: None; CAVH: None
Primaquine	1	4-7/No data	No data	3-4	15 mg (base) q24h	I	No data: 100%	No data: 100%	No data: 100%	Hemo: No data: None; CAPD: No data: None; CAVH: No data: Dose for GFR 10-50

Methemoglobinemia at high doses; intravascular hemolysis in patients with G6PD deficiency.

Drug				Dose		GFR >50	GFR 10–50	GFR <10	Dialysis
Pyrimethamine	15-30	80-100/Unchanged	27	2.9	25-75 mg q24h		100%	100%	100%	Hemo: None; CAPD: None; CAVH: None

Metabolites excreted for weeks after drug stopped. Doses are for treatment of toxoplasmosis. Antimalarial doses are much lower. Reduces renal secretion of creatinine.

For definitions of the abbreviations used in the tables, see page 16.

Antimicrobial Agents (continued)

Drug, Toxicity Notes	Percent Excreted Unchanged %	Half-Life (Normal/ ESRD) h	Plasma Protein Binding %	Volume of Distribution L/kg	Dose for Normal Renal Function	Method	Adjustment for Renal Failure GFR, mL/min >50	10-50	<10	Supplement for Dialysis
Antiparasitic Antibiotics (continued)										
Quinine Marked tissue accumulation.	5-20	3-20/Unchanged	70	0.7-3.7	650 mg q8h	I	q8h	q8-12h	q24h	Hemo: Dose after dialysis CAPD: Dose for GFR <10 CAVH: Dose for GFR 10-50
Trimetrexate Must administer with leucovorin (folinic acid).	5-33	4-22/No data	95	0.6 (10-31L/m²)	45 mg/m² q24h adjust based on hematologic parameters	D	100%	No data: 50-100%	No data: Avoid?	Hemo: No data CAPD: No data CAVH: No data
Antituberculous Antibiotics										
Rifampin Many drug interactions.	15-30	1.5-5.0/1.8-11.0	60-90	0.9	600 mg q24h	D	100%	50-100%	50-100%	Hemo: None CAPD: Dose for GFR <10 CAVH: Dose for GFR <10
Antiviral Agents										
Acyclovir Neurotoxicity in ESRD. Intravenous preparation can cause renal failure if injected rapidly.	40-70	2.1-3.8/20	15-30	0.7	5.0 mg/kg q8h	D,I	5 mg/kg q8h	5 mg/kg q12-24h	2.5 mg/kg q24h	Hemo: Dose after dialysis CAPD: Dose for GFR <10 CAVH: 3.5 mg/kg/d
Amantadine	90	12/500	60	4-5	100 mg q12h	I	q24-48h	q48-72h	q7d	Hemo: None CAPD: None CAVH: Dose for GFR 10-50

Drug					Dose for Normal Renal Function	Method	GFR >50	GFR 10–50	GFR <10	Supplement
Cidofovir	90	2.5/No data	< 6	0.3–0.8	5 mg/kg weekly ×2 (induction); 5 mg/kg every 2 weeks (maintenance)	D	No data: 50–100%	No data: Avoid	No data: Avoid	Hemo: No data CAPD: No data CAVH: Avoid
Dose-limiting nephrotoxicity with proteinuria, glycosuria, renal insufficiency; nephrotoxicity and renal clearance reduced with coadministration of probenecid.										
Delavirdine	5	5.8/No data	98	0.5	400 mg q8h	D	No data: 100%	No data: 100%	No data: 100%	Hemo: No data: None CAPD: No data CAVH: No data: Dose for GFR 10-50
Didanosine	40–69	0.6–1.6/4.5	< 5	1.0	200 mg q12h (125 mg if < 60 kg)	D	q12h	q24h	50% q24h	Hemo: Dose after dialysis CAPD: Dose for GFR <10 CAVH: Dose for GFR <10
Famciclovir	50–65	1.6–2.9/10–22	< 25	1.5	500 mg q8h for herpes zoster; 125 mg q12h for genital herpes	D	100%	q12–48h	50% q48h	Hemo: Dose after dialysis CAPD: No data CAVH: No data: Dose for GFR 10-50
Metabolized to active compound penciclovir.										
Foscarnet	85	3/Prolonged (up to 100)	17	0.3–0.6	40 mg/kg q8h to 90 mg/kg 12h (depends on indication)	D	28 mg/kg q12h	15 mg/kg q24h	6 mg/kg	Hemo: Dose after dialysis CAPD: Dose for GFR <10 CAVH: Dose for GFR 10-50
Nephrotoxic; seizures, hypokalemia, hypocalcemia, hypomagnesemia.										
Ganciclovir	90–100	3.6/30	No data	0.47	5.0 mg/kg q12h	I	q12h	q24–48h	q48–96h	Hemo: Dose after dialysis CAPD: Dose for GFR <10 CAVH: 2.5 mg/kg q24h
Marrow toxicity.										
Ganciclovir-oral					1000 mg q8h	D,I	No data: 1500 mg q24h	No data: 500–1000 mg q24h	No data: 500 mg q48–96h	Hemo: No data: Dose after dialysis CAPD: No data: Dose for GFR <10 CAVH: Not applicable
Indinavir	10	1.8/No data	60	No data	800 mg q8h		No data: 100%	No data: 100%	No data: 100%	Hemo: No data: None CAPD: No data: Dose for GFR < 10 CAVH: No data
Nephrolithiasis; acute renal failure due to crystalluria, tubulointerstitial nephritis.										

For definitions of the abbreviations used in the tables, see page 16.

59

Antimicrobial Agents (continued)

Drug, Toxicity Notes	Percent Excreted Unchanged	Half-Life (Normal/ ESRD)	Plasma Protein Binding	Volume of Distribution	Dose for Normal Renal Function	Adjustment for Renal Failure				Supplement for Dialysis
						Method	GFR, mL/min			
							>50	10-50	<10	
	%	h	%	L/kg						
Antiviral Agents (continued)										
Lamivudine	70-80	5-11/20	36	0.83	150 mg q12h	D,I	100%	50-150 mg q24h (full first dose)	25-50 mg q24h (50 mg first dose)	Hemo: Dose after dialysis CAPD: No data: Dose for GFR < 10 CAVH: Dose for GFR 10-50
Nelfinavir	No data	1.8-3.4/No data	No data	No data	750 mg q8h			No data	No data	Hemo: No data CAPD: No data CAVH: No data
Nevirapine	< 3	40/No data	60	1.2-1.4	200 mg q24h × 14d then q12h	D	No data: 100%	No data: 100%	No data: 100%	Hemo: No data: None CAPD: No data: Dose for GFR < 10 CAVH: No data: Dose for GFR 10-50
May be partially cleared by hemodialysis and peritoneal dialysis.										
Ribavirin	10-40	30-60/No data	0	9-15	200 mg q8h	D	100%	100%	50%	Hemo: Dose after dialysis CAPD: Dose for GFR <10 CAVH: Dose for GFR <10
Half-life data from multiple doses. Loading dose required. Oral absorption 40%.										
Rifabutin	5-10	16-69/Unchanged	71-89	8.2-9.3	300 mg q24h		100%	100%	100%	Hemo: None CAPD: None CAVH: No data: Dose for GFR 10-50

Drug				Dose	Method	GFR >50	GFR 10-50	GFR <10	Dialysis
Ritonavir	3.5	3-5/No data	98-99	0.4	600 mg q12h		No data: 100%	No data: 100%	No data: 100%	Hemo: No data: None CAPD: No data: Dose for GFR < 10 CAVH: No data: Dose for GFR 10-50
Saquinavir	<4	1-2/No data	98	10	600 mg q8h		No data: 100%	No data: 100%	No data: 100%	Hemo: No data: None CAPD: No data: Dose for GFR < 10 CAVH: No data: Dose for GFR 10-50
Stavudine	35-40	1.0-1.4/5.5-8.0	<1	0.5	30-40 mg q12h	D,I	100%	50% q12-24h	50% q24h	Hemo: Dose for GFR <10 after dialysis CAPD: No data CAVH: No data: Dose for GFR 10-50
Valacyclovir	<1				500 mg q12h to 1000 mg q8h (depends on indication)	D,I	100%	full dose q12-24h	0.5 g q24h	Hemo: Dose after dialysis CAPD: Dose for GFR < 10 CAVH: No data: Dose for GFR 10-50
Vidarabine	50	1.5/No data	25	0.7	15 mg/kg infusion q24h	D	100%	100%	75%	Hemo: Infuse after dialysis CAPD: Dose for GFR <10 CAVH: Dose for GFR 10-50

Valacyclovir: Rapidly and extensively converted to acyclovir; bioavailability of valacyclovir is 50-55% versus 10-20% for standard oral acyclovir preparations; other pharmacokinetic variables and toxicities as for acyclovir.

For definitions of the abbreviations used in the tables, see page 16.

Antimicrobial Agents (Continued)

Drug, Toxicity Notes	Percent Excreted Unchanged	Half-Life (Normal/ ESRD)	Plasma Protein Binding	Volume of Distribution	Dose for Normal Renal Function	Method	Adjustment for Renal Failure GFR, mL/min >50	10-50	<10	Supplement for Dialysis
	%	h	%	L/kg						
Antiviral Agents (Continued)										
Zalcitabine	75	1-2/> 8	< 4	0.54	0.75 mg q8h	I,D	100%	q12h	q24h	Hemo: No data: Dose after dialysis CAPD: No data CAVH: No data: Dose for GFR 10-50
Zidovudine Enormous interpatient variation. Metabolite renally excreted.	8-25	1.1-1.4/1.4-3.0	10-30	1.4-3.0	200 mg q8h, 300 mg q12h	D,I	100%	100%	100 mg q8h	Hemo: Dose for GFR <10 CAPD: Dose for GFR <10 CAVH: 100 mg q8h

For definitions of the abbreviations used in the tables, see page 16.

Miscellaneous Agents

Anticonvulsants

Generalized major motor seizures occur in patients with uremia; phenytoin is one of the most frequently used drugs for such seizures. Phenytoin absorption is slow and erratic, its hepatic metabolism is concentration dependent and saturable, and its distribution and elimination vary. In addition, phenytoin protein binding is decreased and distribution volume increased in renal failure. With any given total serum phenytoin level, the concentration of active, free drug will be higher in uremic patients than in patients with normal renal function. Most clinical laboratories measure the total serum drug concentration; thus, a low total phenytoin level in a patient with renal failure should not necessarily be misinterpreted as subtherapeutic.

Physical findings such as nystagmus may be helpful in deciding not to increase the dose. Seizures are also a manifestation of phenytoin excess, and small dosage increases may result in disproportionately large increases in the serum drug level. Dose increments should be small, sufficient time should be allowed for the patient to reach steady-state drug levels, and measurements of free serum phenytoin concentration should be taken frequently in uremic patients who are not responding to therapy.

Nonsteroidal Anti-inflammatory Drugs

Adverse effects of nonsteroidal anti-inflammatory drugs can be the result of either the pharmacologic action of prostaglandin synthesis inhibition or direct hypersensitivity. Prostaglandins are important in maintaining renal vasodilation and ensuring adequate renal blood flow. Nonsteroidal anti-inflammatory drugs are potent inhibitors of renal prostaglandin synthesis, resulting in renal arteriolar constriction, decreased renal blood flow, and a reduced glomerular filtration rate.

Prostaglandins are also important for maintaining fluid and electrolyte homeostasis. Reduction in glomerular filtration allows increased tubular reabsorption. Decreased prostaglandin production increases tubular chloride reabsorption in Henle's loop and increases the effect of antidiuretic hormone on the distal tubule. These effects may lead to salt and water retention. Also, renin generation is diminished. The resultant decrease in plasma aldosterone production can lead to potassium retention and hyperkalemia in patients with decreased renal function. Adverse effects of nonsteroidal anti-inflammatory drugs are more clinically apparent in patients with decreased effective circulating fluid volume. Thus, patients with congestive heart failure, chronic liver disease, chronic renal failure, dehydration, or hemorrhage are at increased risk for adverse effects.

Acute renal failure characterized by proteinuria or the nephrotic syndrome (i.e., hematuria, pyuria, and histologic evidence of immune glomerular injury or interstitial nephritis) is consistent with a hypersensitivity reaction. Discontinuing treatment with the nonsteroidal anti-inflammatory agent results in the gradual disappearance of proteinuria and a return toward normal renal function.

Miscellaneous Agents

Drug, Toxicity Notes	Percent Excreted Unchanged	Half-Life (Normal/ ESRD)	Plasma Protein Binding	Volume of Distribution	Dose for Normal Renal Function	Method	Adjustment for Renal Failure GFR, mL/min			Supplement for Dialysis
							>50	10-50	<10	
	%	h	%	L/kg						
Anticoagulants										
Alteplase (tissue-type plasminogen activator [tPa])	No data	0.5	No data	0.1	60 mg over 1h then 20 mg/h for 2h	D	100%	100%	100%	Hemo: No data CAPD: No data CAVH: Dose for GFR 10-50
Anistreplase	No data	1.2	No data	0.08	30 U over 2-5 min	D	100%	100%	100%	Hemo: No data CAPD: No data CAVH: Dose for GFR 10-50
Dipyridamole	No data	12/No data	99	2.4	50 mg tid	D	100%	100%	100%	Hemo: No data CAPD: No data CAVH: Not applicable
Heparin Half-life increases with dose.	None	0.3-2/Unchanged	> 90	0.06-0.1	75 U/kg load then 0.5 U/kg/min	D	100%	100%	100%	Hemo: None CAPD: None CAVH: Dose for GFR 10-50
Iloprost	No data	0.3-0.5/Unchanged	No data	0.7	0.5-2.0 ng/kg/min for 5-12h	D	100%	100%	50%	Hemo: No data CAPD: No data CAVH: Dose for GFR 10-50
Indobufen	< 15	6-7/27-33	>99	0.18-0.21	100-200 mg bid	D	100%	50%	25%	Hemo: No data CAPD: No data CAVH: Not applicable

For definitions of the abbreviations used in the tables, see page 16.

Miscellaneous Agents (Continued)

Drug, Toxicity Notes	Percent Excreted Unchanged	Half-Life (Normal/ ESRD)	Plasma Protein Binding	Volume of Distribution	Dose for Normal Renal Function	Method	Adjustment for Renal Failure GFR, mL/min >50	Adjustment for Renal Failure GFR, mL/min 10-50	Adjustment for Renal Failure GFR, mL/min <10	Supplement for Dialysis
	%	h	%	L/kg						
Anticoagulants (Continued)										
Low-molecular-weight heparin	No data	2.2-6.0/4-10	No data	0.06-0.13	30-40 mg bid	D	100%	100%	50%	Hemo: No data CAPD: No data CAVH: Dose for GFR 10-50
Streptokinase	None	0.6-1.5/No data	No data	0.02-0.08	250 000 U load then 100 000 U/h	D	100%	100%	100%	Hemo: Not applicable CAPD: Not applicable CAVH: Dose for GFR 10-50
Sulfinpyrazone Acute renal failure. Uricosuric effect at low GFR.	25-50	2.2-5.0/Unchanged	> 95	0.06	200 mg bid	D	100%	100%	Avoid	Hemo: None CAPD: None CAVH: Dose for GFR 10-50
Sulotroban	52-62	0.7-3/9-39	No data	0.7-0.8	No data	D	50%	30%	10%	Hemo: No data CAPD: No data CAVH: No data
Ticlopidine	2	24-33/No data	98	No data	250 mg bid	D	100%	100%	100%	Hemo: No data CAPD: No data CAVH: Dose for GFR 10-50
Tranexamic acid	90	1.5/No data	3	No data	25 mg/kg tid-qid	D	50%	25%	10%	Hemo: No data CAPD: No data CAVH: No data

Urokinase	No data	No data	No data	No data	4400 U/kg load then 4400 U/kg qh	D	No data	No data	No data	Hemo: No data CAPD: No data CAVH: Dose for GFR 10-50
Warfarin	None	34-45/Unchanged	99	0.15	10-15 mg load then 2-10 mg q24h	D	100%	100%	100%	Hemo: None CAPD: None CAVH: None
Follow prothrombin time. Decreased protein binding in uremia.										

Anticonvulsants

Carbamazepine	2-3	25-65 single; 12-17 chronic/Unchanged	75	0.8-1.6	200 mg bid to 1200 mg q24h	D	100%	100%	100%	Hemo: None CAPD: None CAVH: None
Increase antidiuretic hormone secretion.										
Ethosuximide	17-40	35-55/Unchanged	10	0.6-0.9	500-1500 mg q24h	D	100%	100%	100%	Hemo: None CAPD: No data CAVH: No data
Gabapentin	90	5-7/132	Unbound	0.7	300-600 mg tid	D,I	400 mg tid	300 mg q12-24h	300 mg qod	Hemo: 300 mg load, then 200-300 after hemodialysis CAPD: 300 mg qod CAVH: Dose for GFR 10-50
Lamotrigine	10	25-30/Unchanged	0.55	0.9-1.3	50 mg q12-24h (initially); 100-500 mg q24h (maintenance)	D	100%	100%	100%	Hemo: No data CAPD: No data CAVH: Dose for GFR 10-50
Oxcarbazepine	< 1	10-25/Unchanged	40	0.7-0.8	200-400 mg tid	D	100%	100%	100%	Hemo: No data CAPD: No data CAVH: No data
Phenytoin	2	24/Unchanged	90	1	1000 mg load then 300-400 mg q24h	D	100%	100%	100%	Hemo: None CAPD: None CAVH: None
Measure free levels. Protein binding decreased and distribution volume increased in renal failure. Folate deficiency. Interstitial nephritis.										

For definitions of the abbreviations used in the tables, see page 16.

Miscellaneous Agents (Continued)

Drug, Toxicity Notes	Percent Excreted Unchanged	Half-Life (Normal/ ESRD)	Plasma Protein Binding	Volume of Distribution	Dose for Normal Renal Function	Method	>50	10-50	<10	Supplement for Dialysis
	%	h	%	L/kg						
Anticonvulsants (Continued)										
Primidone	40	5-15/Unchanged	20-30	0.4-1	250-500 mg qid	I	q8h	q8-12h	q12-24h	Hemo: 1/3 dose CAPD: No data CAVH: No data
Partially converted to phenobarbital and other metabolites with long half-life. Excessive sedation. Nystagmus. Folate deficiency.										
Sodium valproate	3-7	6-15/Unchanged	90	0.19-0.23	15-60 mg/kg q24h	D	100%	100%	100%	Hemo: None CAPD: None CAVH: None
Decreased protein binding in uremia. Concurrent phenytoin, phenobarbital, and primidone shorten half-life.										
Topiramate	70-80	19-23/48-60	9-17	0.6-0.8	100-400 mg q12-24h	D	100%	50%	25%	Hemo: No data CAPD: No data CAVH: Dose for GFR 10-50
Trimethadione	None	12-24/No data	None	No data	300-600 mg tid-qid	I	q8h	q8-12h	q12-24h	Hemo: No data CAPD: No data CAVH: Dose for GFR 10-50
Active metabolites with long half-life in ESRD. Nephrotic syndrome.										
Vigabatrin	70	5-7/13-15	None	0.8	1-2 g bid	D	100%	50%	25%	Hemo: No data CAPD: No data CAVH: Dose for GFR 10-50

Antihistamines

H₁ Antagonists
May cause excessive sedation in ESRD.

Acrivastine	60	1.4-2.1/No data	50	0.6-0.7	8.0 mg tid or qid	D	100%	50%	50%	Hemo: No data CAPD: No data CAVH: No data
Astemizole	None	20 d/Unchanged	97	No data	10 mg q24h	D	100%	100%	100%	Hemo: No data CAPD: No data CAVH: Not applicable
Brompheniramine	3	6/No data	No data	12	4.0 mg q4-6h	D	100%	100%	100%	Hemo: No data CAPD: No data CAVH: Not applicable
Cetirizine	60-70	7-10/20	93	0.4-0.6	5-20 mg q24h	D	100%	50%	25%	Hemo: None CAPD: No data CAVH: Not applicable
Chlorpheniramine	20	14-24/No data	72	6-12	4.0 mg q4-6h	D	100%	100%	100%	Hemo: None CAPD: No data CAVH: Not applicable
Diphenhydramine	2	3.4-9.3/No data	80	3.3-6.8	25 mg tid-qid	D	100%	100%	100%	Hemo: None CAPD: None CAVH: None
Erbastine	40	13-16/23-26	98	1-2	10 mg q24h	D	100%	50%	50%	Hemo: No data CAPD: No data CAVH: Dose for GFR 10-50

Diphenhydramine: Anticholinergic effects may cause urinary retention.

For definitions of the abbreviations used in the tables, see page 16.

69

Miscellaneous Agents (Continued)

Drug, Toxicity Notes	Percent Excreted Unchanged	Half-Life (Normal/ ESRD)	Plasma Protein Binding	Volume of Distribution	Dose for Normal Renal Function	Method	Adjustment for Renal Failure GFR, mL/min			Supplement for Dialysis
							>50	10-50	<10	
	%	h	%	L/kg						

H₁ Antagonists (Continued)

Antihistamines (Continued)

Drug, Toxicity Notes	Percent Excreted Unchanged	Half-Life (Normal/ESRD)	Plasma Protein Binding	Volume of Distribution	Dose for Normal Renal Function	Method	>50	10-50	<10	Supplement for Dialysis
Fexofenadine	10	14/19-25	70	5-6	60 mg bid	I	q12h	q12-24h	q24h	Hemo: No data CAPD: No data CAVH: Dose for GFR 10-50
Flunarizine	None	17-18 d/No data	99	43-78	10-20 mg q24h	D	100%	100%	100%	Hemo: None CAPD: None CAVH: None
Hydroxyzine Accumulates in ESRD.	None	14-20/No data	No data	19.5	50-100 mg qid	D	100%	50%	50%	Hemo: 1 CAPD: 1 CAVH: 1
Orphenadrine	8	16/No data	No data	No data	100 mg bid	D	100%	100%	100%	Hemo: No data CAPD: No data CAVH: Not applicable
Oxatomide	None	20/No data	91	No data	No data	D	100%	100%	100%	Hemo: None CAPD: None CAVH: Not applicable
Promethazine	None	12/No data	93	13.5	12.5-25 mg qd-qid	D	100%	100%	100%	Hemo: None CAPD: None CAVH: 1

Drug					Dose					
Terfenadine Causes torsades de pointes.	None	16-23/No data	97	No data	60 mg bid	D	100%	100%	100%	Hemo: None CAPD: None CAVH: Not applicable
Tripelennamine	No data	3.0-4.5/No data	No data	10	25-50 mg tid-qid	D	No data	No data	No data	Hemo: No data CAPD: No data CAVH: Not applicable
Triprolidine	No data	5/No data	No data	No data	2.5 mg q4-6h	D	No data	No data	No data	Hemo: No data CAPD: No data CAVH: Not applicable

H₂ Antagonists

Drug					Dose					
Cimetidine Increases serum creatinine and decreases creatinine clearance by inhibition of creatinine secretion. Mental confusion with renal or hepatic disease. Acute renal failure.	50-70	1.5-2.0/5	20	0.8-1.3	400 mg bid or 400-800 mg qhs	D	100%	50%	25%	Hemo: None CAPD: None CAVH: Dose for GFR 10-50
Famotidine	65-80	2.5-4.0/12-19	15-22	0.8-1.4	20-40 mg qhs	D	50%	25%	10%	Hemo: None CAPD: None CAVH: Dose for GFR 10-50
Nizatidine	10-15	1.3-1.6/5.3-8.5	28-35	0.8-1.3	150-300 mg qhs	D	75%	50%	25%	Hemo: No data CAPD: No data CAVH: Dose for GFR 10-50
Ranitidine	80	1.5-3.0/6-9	15	1.2-1.8	150-300 mg qhs	D	75%	50%	25%	Hemo: 1/2 dose CAPD: None CAVH: Dose for GFR 10-50

For definitions of the abbreviations used in the tables, see page 16.

Miscellaneous Agents (Continued)

Drug, Toxicity Notes	Percent Excreted Unchanged	Half-Life (Normal/ ESRD)	Plasma Protein Binding	Volume of Distribution	Dose for Normal Renal Function	Adjustment for Renal Failure				Supplement for Dialysis
						Method	GFR, mL/min			
							>50	10-50	<10	
	%	h	%	L/kg						
Antineoplastic Agents										
Myelosuppressive and may aggravate uremic predisposition to hemorrhage and infection.										
Altretamine	< 10	7/No data	No data	No data	150-200 mg/m^2	D	No data	No data	No data	Hemo: No data CAPD: No data CAVH: No data
Azathioprine 6-Mercaptopurine is active metabolite.	< 2	0.16-1/Increased	20	0.55-0.8	1.5-2.5 mg/kg q24h	D	100%	75%	50%	Hemo: Supplement 0.25 mg/kg CAPD: No data CAVH: Dose for GFR 10-50
Bleomycin Drug accumulation predisposes to pulmonary fibrosis. Hypertension and dysuria.	60	9/20	No data	0.3	10-20 U/m^2	D	100%	75%	50%	Hemo: None CAPD: No data CAVH: Dose for GFR 10-50
Busulfan Hemorrhagic cystitis.	0.5-3	2.5-3.4/No data	3-15	1	4-8 mg q24h	D	100%	100%	100%	Hemo: No data CAPD: No data CAVH: Dose for GFR 10-50
Carboplatin	50-75	6/Increased	15-24	0.23-0.28	360 mg/m^2	D	100%	50%	25%	Hemo: 1/2 dose CAPD: No data CAVH: Dose for GFR 10-50
Carmustine	No data	1.5/No data	No data	3.3	150-200 mg/m^2	D	No data	No data	Avoid	Hemo: No data CAPD: No data CAVH: No data

Chlorambucil	No data	1/No data	No data	0.86	0.1 mg/kg q24h	D	No data	No data	No data	Hemo: No data CAPD: No data CAVH: No data
Cisplatin	27-45	0.3-0.5/No data	90	0.5	20-50 mg/m² q24h	D	100%	75%	50%	Hemo: Yes CAPD: No data CAVH: Dose for GFR 10-50
Nephrotoxic. Toxicity reduced by pretreatment hydration. Renal Mg^{++} wasting.										
Cladribine	No data	7-14/No data	No data	50-80	0.1 mg/kg q24h	D	No data	No data	No data	Hemo: No data CAPD: No data CAVH: No data
Cyclophosphamide	10-15	4.0-7.5/10	14-20	0.5-1	1-5 mg/kg q24h	D	100%	100%	75%	Hemo: 1/2 dose CAPD: No data CAVH: Dose for GFR 10-50
Hemorrhagic cystitis. Bladder fibrosis and bladder cancer. Increased antidiuretic hormone secretion.										
Cytarabine	6	0.5-3/Unchanged	13	2.6	100-200 mg/m²	D	100%	100%	100%	Hemo: No data CAPD: No data CAVH: Dose for GFR 10-50
Daunorubicin	None	18-27/No data	No data	No data	30-45 mg/m²	D	100%	100%	100%	Hemo: No data CAPD: No data CAVH: No data
Doxorubicin	< 15	35/Unchanged	80-85	21.5	60-75 mg/m² q24h	D	100%	100%	100%	Hemo: None CAPD: No data CAVH: Dose for GFR 10-50
Acute renal failure and nephrotic syndrome.										
Epirubicin	< 15	35/35	80-85	10-40	50 mg/m² q24h	D	100%	100%	100%	Hemo: None CAPD: No data CAVH: Dose for GFR 10-50
Etoposide	20-60	4-18/19	74-94	0.17-0.5	35-100 mg/m² q24h	D	100%	75%	50%	Hemo: None CAPD: No data CAVH: Dose for GFR 10-50

For definitions of the abbreviations used in the tables, see page 16.

Miscellaneous Agents (Continued)

Drug, Toxicity Notes	Percent Excreted Unchanged	Half-Life (Normal/ ESRD)	Plasma Protein Binding	Volume of Distribution	Dose for Normal Renal Function	Adjustment for Renal Failure Method	Adjustment for Renal Failure GFR, mL/min >50	Adjustment for Renal Failure GFR, mL/min 10-50	Adjustment for Renal Failure GFR, mL/min <10	Supplement for Dialysis
	%	h	%	L/kg						
Antineoplastic Agents (Continued)										
Fludarabine	50	7-12/24	No data	5-40	25-50 mg/m² q24h	D	100%	75%	50%	Hemo: No data CAPD: No data CAVH: Dose for GFR 10-50
Fluorouracil	< 5	0.1/Unchanged	10	0.25-0.5	12 mg/kg q24h	D	100%	100%	100%	Hemo: Give 1/2 dose CAPD: No data CAVH: Dose for GFR 10-50
Flutamide Gynecomastia, antiantidrogenic.	40	4-6/No data	No data	No data	150 mg q8h	D	100%	100%	100%	Hemo: No data CAPD: No data CAVH: No data
Hydroxyurea	>50	No data	No data	0.5	20-30 mg/kg q24h	D	100%	50%	20%	Hemo: No data CAPD: No data CAVH: Dose for GFR 10-50
Idarubicin	< 10	36-70/No data	No data	No data	10-12 mg/m² IV for 3-4 days	D	No data	No data	No data	Hemo: No data CAPD: No data CAVH: No data
Ifosfamide Associated with Fanconi syndrome and renal dysfunction.	15	4-10/No data	No data	0.4-0.64	1.2 g/m²	D	100%	100%	75%	Hemo: No data CAPD: No data CAVH: Dose for GFR 10-50
Melphalan	12	1.1-1.4/4-6	90	0.6-0.75	6.0 mg q24h	D	100%	75%	50%	Hemo: No data CAPD: No data CAVH: Dose for GFR 10-50

Drug				Dose		>50	10-50	<10	Supplement for dialysis
Methotrexate	80-90	8-12/Increased	45-50	0.76	5-10 mg/wk (rheumatoid arthritis) 15 m/d to 12 g/m² (cancer)	D	100%	50%	Avoid	Hemo: Give 1/2 dose CAPD: None CAVH: Dose for GFR 10-50
		Nephrotoxicity decreased by urinary alkalinization and forced diuresis.								
Mitomycin C	No data	0.5-1/No data	No data	0.5	20 mg/m² q6-8wk	D	100%	100%	75%	Hemo: No data CAPD: No data CAVH: No data
		Nephrotoxicity. Hemolytic uremic syndrome.								
Mitoxantrone	< 10	23-40/No data	75	200-300	10-15 mg/m² qd-qwk	D	100%	100%	100%	Hemo: No data CAPD: No data CAVH: Dose for GFR 10-50
Nitrosoureas	> 50	Short/No data	No data	No data	Varies	D	100%	75%	25%-50%	Hemo: None CAPD: No data CAVH: No data
		Prototype methyl CCNU. Metabolites with variable $T_{1/2}$. Irreversible toxicity at dose >1500 mg/m².								
Paclitaxel	5-10	9-30/No data	No data	30-60	100-200 mg/m²	D	100%	100%	100%	Hemo: No data CAPD: No data CAVH: Dose for GFR 10-50
Plicamycin	> 50	2/No data	< 10	No data	25-30 µg/kg q24h	D	100%	75%	50%	Hemo: No data CAPD: No data CAVH: No data
		Cumulative nephrotoxicity. Acute renal failure. Decrease serum Ca++, K+, phosphate.								
Streptozocin	None	0.25/No data	0.5	No data	500 mg/m² q24h	D	100%	75%	50%	Hemo: No data CAPD: No data CAVH: No data
		Nephrotoxic. Proteinuria. Low serum phosphate. Renal tubular acidosis.								
Tamoxifen	None	18/No data	> 98	20	10-20 mg bid	D	100%	100%	100%	Hemo: No data CAPD: No data CAVH: Dose for GFR 10-50
		Hot flashes, nausea, vomiting.								
Teniposide	4-14	6-10/No data	99	0.2-0.7	50-250 mg/m²	D	100%	100%	100%	Hemo: None CAPD: None CAVH: Dose for GFR 10-50

For definitions of the abbreviations used in the tables, see page 16.

Miscellaneous Agents (Continued)

Drug, Toxicity Notes	Percent Excreted Unchanged	Half-Life (Normal/ ESRD)	Plasma Protein Binding	Volume of Distribution	Dose for Normal Renal Function	Method	>50	10-50	<10	Supplement for Dialysis
	%	h	%	L/kg						
				Antineoplastic Agents (Continued)						
Topotecan	40	4-6/Prolonged	No data	40	5-20 mg/m² every 1-3 weeks	D	75%	50%	25%	Hemo: No data CAPD: No data CAVH: Dose for GFR 10-50
Vinblastine	None	1.0-1.5/No data	75	13-40	3.7 mg/m²	D	100%	100%	100%	Hemo: No data CAPD: No data CAVH: Dose for GFR 10-50
Vinca alkaloids may increase antidiuretic hormone secretion. Vd increases with time due to avid tissue binding.										
Vincristine	12	1.0-2.5/No data	75	5-11	1.4 mg/m²	D	100%	100%	100%	Hemo: No data CAPD: No data CAVH: Dose for GFR 10-50
Vinorelbine	< 20	20-40/No data	15	75	5-8 mg/m² q24h	D	100%	100%	100%	Hemo: No data CAPD: No data CAVH: Dose for GFR 10-50
				Antiparkinson Agents						
Require careful titration of dose according to clinical response.										
Carbidopa	30	2/No data	No data	No data	1 tab tid to 6 tabs daily	D	100%	100%	100%	Hemo: No data CAPD: No data CAVH: No data

Antithyroid Drugs

Drug	% Protein Binding	Half-Life (Normal/ESRD)	% Excreted	Vd	Dose	Method	GFR > 50	GFR 10-50	GFR < 10	Supplement
Levodopa	None	0.8-1.6/No data	5-8	0.9-1.6	250-500 mg bid to 8 g q24h	D	100%	50-100%	50-100%	Hemo: No data CAPD: No data CAVH: Dose for GFR 10-50
Methimazole	7	3-6/Unchanged	None	0.6	5-20 mg tid	D	100%	100%	100%	Hemo: No data CAPD: No data CAVH: Dose for GFR 10-50
Propylthiouracil	< 10	1-2/Unchanged	80	0.3-0.4	100 mg tid	D	100%	100%	100%	Hemo: No data CAPD: No data CAVH: Dose for GFR 10-50

Levodopa: Active and inactive metabolites excreted in urine. Active metabolites with long $T_{1/2}$ in ESRD.

Arthritis and Gout Agents

Drug	% Protein Binding	Half-Life (Normal/ESRD)	% Excreted	Vd	Dose	Method	GFR > 50	GFR 10-50	GFR < 10	Supplement
Allopurinol	30	2-8/Unchanged	< 5	0.5	300 mg q24h	D	75%	50%	25%	Hemo: 1/2 dose CAPD: No data CAVH: Dose for GFR 10-50
Auranofin	50	70-80 d/No data	60	No data	6.0 mg q24h	D	50%	Avoid	Avoid	Hemo: None CAPD: None CAVH: None
Colchicine	5-17	4/19-50	31	4	Acute: 2 mg then 0.5 mg q6h Chronic: 0.5-1.0 mg q24h	D	100%	50-100%	25%	Hemo: None CAPD: No data CAVH: Dose for GFR 10-50
Gold sodium thiomalate	60-90	250 d/No data	95	5-9	25-50 mg	D	50%	Avoid	Avoid	Hemo: None CAPD: None CAVH: Avoid
Penicillamine	40	1.5-3.0/Increased	80	No data	250-1000 mg q24h	D	100%	Avoid	Avoid	Hemo: 1/3 dose CAPD: No data CAVH: Dose for GFR 10-50

Allopurinol: Interstitial nephritis. Rare xanthine stones. Renal excretion of active metabolite with $T_{1/2}$ of 25 hours in normal renal function; $T_{1/2}$ one week in patients with ESRD. Exfoliative dermatitis.

Auranofin: Proteinuria and nephrotic syndrome.

Colchicine: Avoid prolonged use if GFR < 50 mL/min.

Gold sodium thiomalate: Proteinuria; nephrotic syndrome; membranous nephritis.

Penicillamine: Nephrotic syndrome.

For definitions of the abbreviations used in the tables, see page 16.

Miscellaneous Agents (Continued)

Drug, Toxicity Notes	Percent Excreted Unchanged	Half-Life (Normal/ ESRD)	Plasma Protein Binding	Volume of Distribution	Dose for Normal Renal Function	Adjustment for Renal Failure				Supplement for Dialysis
						Method	GFR, mL/min			
							>50	10-50	<10	
	%	h	%	L/kg						

Arthritis and Gout Agents (Continued)

Drug, Toxicity Notes	Percent Excreted Unchanged	Half-Life (Normal/ ESRD)	Plasma Protein Binding	Volume of Distribution	Dose for Normal Renal Function	Method	>50	10-50	<10	Supplement for Dialysis
Probenecid Ineffective at decreased GFR.	< 2	5-8/Unchanged	85-95	0.15	500 mg bid	D	100%	Avoid	Avoid	Hemo: Avoid CAPD: No data CAVH: Avoid

Arthritis and Gout Agents: Nonsteroidal Anti-inflammatory Drugs

May decrease renal function. Decrease platelet aggregation. Nephrotic syndrome. Interstitial nephritis. Hyperkalemia. Sodium retention.

Drug, Toxicity Notes	Percent Excreted Unchanged	Half-Life (Normal/ ESRD)	Plasma Protein Binding	Volume of Distribution	Dose for Normal Renal Function	Method	>50	10-50	<10	Supplement for Dialysis
Diclofenac	< 1	1-2/Unchanged	> 99	0.12-0.17	25-75 mg bid	D	50-100%	25-50%	25%	Hemo: None CAPD: None CAVH: Dose for GFR 10-50
Diflunisal	< 3	5-20/62	> 99	0.1-0.13	250-500 mg bid	D	100%	50%	50%	Hemo: None CAPD: None CAVH: Dose for GFR 10-50
Etodolac	Negligible	5-7/Unchanged	> 99	0.4	200 mg bid	D	100%	100%	100%	Hemo: None CAPD: None CAVH: Dose for GFR 10-50
Fenoprofen	30	2-3/Unchanged	> 99	0.1	300-600 mg qid	D	100%	100%	100%	Hemo: None CAPD: None CAVH: Dose for GFR 10-50

Drug		Half-life (Normal/ESRD)		Vd	Dose	Method	GFR >50	GFR 10-50	GFR <10	Dialysis
Flurbiprofen	20	3-5/Unchanged	99	0.1-0.2	100 mg bid-tid	D	100%	100%	100%	Hemo: None CAPD: None CAVH: Dose for GFR 10-50
Ibuprofen	1	2-3.2/Unchanged	99	0.15-0.17	800 mg tid	D	100%	100%	100%	Hemo: None CAPD: None CAVH: Dose for GFR 10-50
Indomethacin	30	4-12/Unchanged	99	0.12	25-50 mg tid	D	100%	100%	100%	Hemo: None CAPD: None CAVH: Dose for GFR 10-50
Ketoprofen	<1	1.5-4/Unchanged	99	0.11	25-75 mg tid	D	100%	100%	100%	Hemo: None CAPD: None CAVH: Dose for GFR 10-50
Ketorolac Acute hearing loss in ESRD.	30-60	4-6/10	>99	0.13-0.25	30-60 mg load then 15-30 mg q6h	D	100%	50%	25-50%	Hemo: None CAPD: None CAVH: Dose for GFR 10-50
Meclofenamic acid	2-4	3/Unchanged	>99	No data	50-100 mg tid-qid	D	100%	100%	100%	Hemo: None CAPD: None CAVH: Dose for GFR 10-50
Mefenamic acid	<6	3-4/Unchanged	No data	No data	250 mg qid	D	100%	100%	100%	Hemo: None CAPD: None CAVH: Dose for GFR 10-50
Nabumetone	<1	24/Unchanged	>99	0.11	1.0-2.0 g q24h	D	100%	50-100%	50-100%	Hemo: None CAPD: None CAVH: Dose for GFR 10-50
Naproxen	<1	12-15/Unchanged	99	0.1	500 mg bid	D	100%	100%	100%	Hemo: None CAPD: None CAVH: Dose for GFR 10-50
Oxaproxin	<1	50-60/Unchanged	>99	0.2	1200 mg q24h	D	100%	100%	100%	Hemo: None CAPD: None CAVH: Dose for GFR 10-50

For definitions of the abbreviations used in the tables, see page 16.

Miscellaneous Agents (Continued)

Drug, Toxicity Notes	Percent Excreted Unchanged	Half-Life (Normal/ESRD)	Plasma Protein Binding	Volume of Distribution	Dose for Normal Renal Function	Method	Adjustment for Renal Failure GFR, mL/min >50	10-50	<10	Supplement for Dialysis
	%	h	%	L/kg						
Arthritis and Gout Agents: Nonsteroidal Anti-inflammatory Drugs (Continued)										
Phenylbutazone	1	50-100/Unchanged	99	.09-0.17	100 mg tid-qid	D	100%	100%	100%	Hemo: None CAPD: None CAVH: Dose for GFR 10-50
Piroxicam	10	45-55/Unchanged	> 99	0.12-0.15	20 mg q24h	D	100%	100%	100%	Hemo: None CAPD: None CAVH: Dose for GFR 10-50
Sulindac Active sulfide metabolite in ESRD.	7	8-16/Unchanged	95	No data	200 mg bid	D	100%	100%	100%	Hemo: None CAPD: None CAVH: Dose for GFR 10-50
Tolmetin	15	1.0-1.5/Unchanged	> 99	0.1-0.14	400 mg tid	D	100%	100%	100%	Hemo: None CAPD: None CAVH: Dose for GFR 10-50
Bronchodilators										
Albuterol	51-64	2-4/4	7	2.0-2.5	2-4 mg tid to qid	D	100%	75%	50%	Hemo: No data CAPD: No data CAVH: Dose for GFR 10-50
Dyphylline	85	1.8-2.3/12	< 3	0.8	15 mg/kg q24h	D	75%	50%	25%	Hemo: 1/3 dose CAPD: No data CAVH: Dose for GFR 10-50

Drug	Percent Excreted	Half-Life (Normal/ESRD)	Protein Binding (%)	Vd (L/kg)	Dose	Method	GFR >50	GFR 10–50	GFR <10	Supplement for Dialysis
Ipratropium	No data	1.6/No data	No data	4.6	2 inhalations qid	D	100%	100%	100%	Hemo: None / CAPD: None / CAVH: Dose for GFR 10-50
Metaproterenol	No data	2-6/No data	10	7.6	2-3 inhalations q3-4h	D	100%	100%	100%	Hemo: No data / CAPD: No data / CAVH: Dose for GFR 10-50
Terbutaline	55-60	3/No data	15-25	0.9-1.5	2.5-5 mg tid	D	100%	50%	Avoid	Hemo: No data / CAPD: No data / CAVH: Dose for GFR 10-50
Large first-dose effect. Avoid parenteral doses in ESRD. Oral doses unchanged.										
Theophylline	None	4-12/Unchanged	55	0.4-0.7	6.0 mg/kg load then 9 mg/kg q24h	D	100%	100%	100%	Hemo: 1/2 dose / CAPD: No data / CAVH: Dose for GFR 10-50
May exacerbate uremic gastrointestinal symptoms.										
Bronchodilators: Leukotriene Inhibitors										
Zafirlukast	<5	10/Unchanged	99	No data	20 mg bid	D	100%	100%	100%	Hemo: No data / CAPD: No data / CAVH: Dose for GFR 10-50
Zileuton	<10	2.3/Unchanged	>90	2.3	600 mg qid	D	100%	100%	100%	Hemo: No data / CAPD: No data / CAVH: Dose for GFR 10-50
Corticosteroids										
May aggravate azotemia, Na$^+$ retention, glucose intolerance, and hypertension.										
Betamethasone	5	5.5/No data	65	1.4	0.5-9.0 mg q24h	D	100%	100%	100%	Hemo: No data / CAPD: No data / CAVH: Dose for GFR 10-50

For definitions of the abbreviations used in the tables, see page 16.

Miscellaneous Agents (Continued)

Drug, Toxicity Notes	Percent Excreted Unchanged	Half-Life (Normal/ ESRD)	Plasma Protein Binding	Volume of Distribution	Dose for Normal Renal Function	Adjustment for Renal Failure Method	GFR, mL/min >50	GFR, mL/min 10-50	GFR, mL/min <10	Supplement for Dialysis
	%	h	%	L/kg						
					Corticosteroids (Continued)					
Budesonide	None	2.0-2.7/No data	88	4.3	No data	D	100%	100%	100%	Hemo: No data CAPD: No data CAVH: Dose for GFR 10-50
Cortisone	None	0.5-2/3.5	90	No data	25-500 mg q24h	D	100%	100%	100%	Hemo: None CAPD: No data CAVH: Dose for GFR 10-50
Dexamethasone	8	3-4/No data	70	0.8-1	0.75-9.0 mg q24h	D	100%	100%	100%	Hemo: No data CAPD: No data CAVH: Dose for GFR 10-50
Hydrocortisone	None	1.5-2.0/No data	No data	No data	20-500 mg q24h	D	100%	100%	100%	Hemo: No data CAPD: No data CAVH: Dose for GFR 10-50
Methylprednisolone	<10	1.9-6.0/Unchanged	40-60	1.2-1.5	4-48 mg q24h	D	100%	100%	100%	Hemo: Yes CAPD: No data CAVH: Dose for GFR 10-50
Prednisolone	34	2.5-3.5/Unchanged	Up to 80	2.2	5-60 mg q24h	D	100%	100%	100%	Hemo: Yes CAPD: No data CAVH: Dose for GFR 10-50
Prednisone	34	2.5-3.5/Unchanged	Up to 80	2.2	5-60 mg q24h	D	100%	100%	100%	Hemo: None CAPD: No data CAVH: Dose for GFR 10-50

Triamcinolone	No data	1.9-6.0/Unchanged	No data	1.4-2.1	4-48 mg q24h	D	100%	100%	100%	Hemo: No data CAPD: No data CAVH: Dose for GFR 10-50

Hypoglycemic Agents (Oral)

Avoid all oral hypoglycemic agents on CRRT.

Drug										Dialysis
Acarbose	35	3-9/Prolonged	15	0.32	50-200 mg tid	D	50-100%	Avoid	Avoid	Hemo: No data / CAPD: No data / CAVH: Avoid
Acetohexamide	None	1.0-1.3/Prolonged	65-90	0.21	250-1500 mg q24h	I	Avoid	Avoid	Avoid	Hemo: No data / CAPD: None / CAVH: Avoid

Diuretic effect. May falsely elevate serum creatinine. Active metabolite has $T_{1/2}$ of 5-8 hours in healthy subjects and is eliminated by the kidney. Prolonged hypoglycemia in azotemic patients.

Chlorpropamide	47	24-48/50-200	88-96	0.09-0.27	100-500 mg q24h	D	50%	Avoid	Avoid	Hemo: None / CAPD: None / CAVH: Avoid

Impairs water excretion. Prolonged hypoglycemia in azotemic patients.

Glibornuride	No data	5-12/No data	95	0.25	12.5-100 mg q24h	D	No data	No data	No data	Hemo: No data / CAPD: No data / CAVH: Avoid
Gliclazide	<20	8-11/No data	85-95	0.24	80-320 mg q24h	D	50-100%	Avoid	Avoid	Hemo: No data / CAPD: No data / CAVH: Avoid
Glipizide	4.5-7	3-7/No data	97	0.13-0.16	2.5-15 mg q24h	D	100%	50%	50%	Hemo: No data / CAPD: No data / CAVH: Avoid
Glyburide	50	1.4-2.9/No data	99	0.16-0.3	1.25-20 mg q24h	D	No data	Avoid	Avoid	Hemo: None / CAPD: None / CAVH: Avoid

For definitions of the abbreviations used in the tables, see page 16.

Miscellaneous Agents (Continued)

Drug, Toxicity Notes	Percent Excreted Unchanged %	Half-Life (Normal/ ESRD) h	Plasma Protein Binding %	Volume of Distribution L/kg	Dose for Normal Renal Function	Adjustment for Renal Failure			Supplement for Dialysis
						Method	>50	GFR, mL/min 10-50	<10	

Hypoglycemic Agents (Oral) (Continued)

Drug, Toxicity Notes	Percent Excreted Unchanged %	Half-Life (Normal/ ESRD) h	Plasma Protein Binding %	Volume of Distribution L/kg	Dose for Normal Renal Function	Method	>50	10-50	<10	Supplement for Dialysis
Metformin Lactic acidosis.	90-100	1-5/Prolonged	Negligible	1-4	500-850 mg bid	D	50%	25%	Avoid	Hemo: No data CAPD: No data CAVH: Avoid
Tolazamide Diuretic effects.	7	4-7/No data	94	No data	100-250 mg q24h	D	100%	100%	100%	Hemo: No data CAPD: No data CAVH: Avoid
Tolbutamide May impair water excretion.	None	4-6/Unchanged	95-97	0.1-0.15	1-2 g q24h	D	100%	100%	100%	Hemo: None CAPD: None CAVH: Avoid

Hypoglycemic Agents (Parenteral)

Dosage guided by blood glucose levels.

Drug, Toxicity Notes	Percent Excreted Unchanged %	Half-Life (Normal/ ESRD) h	Plasma Protein Binding %	Volume of Distribution L/kg	Dose for Normal Renal Function	Method	>50	10-50	<10	Supplement for Dialysis
Insulin Renal metabolism of insulin decreases with azotemia.	None	2-4/Increased	5	0.15	Variable	D	100%	75%	50%	Hemo: None CAPD: None CAVH: Dose for GFR 10-50
Lispro insulin Avoid all oral hypoglycemic agents on CRRT.	No data	1/Prolonged	No data	0.26-0.36	Variable	D	100%	75%	50%	Hemo: None CAPD: None CAVH: None

Hypolipidemic Agents

Drug						50-100%	25-50%	Avoid	
Bezafibrate	50	2.1/7.8-20	95	0.24-0.35	200 mg bid-qid 400 mg SR q24h	D	50-100%	25-50%	Avoid	Hemo: No data / CAPD: No data / CAVH: Dose for GFR 10-50
Cholestyramine Hyperchloremic acidosis.	None	Not absorbed	None	None	4.0 g q4-6h	D	100%	100%	100%	Hemo: None / CAPD: None / CAVH: Dose for GFR 10-50
Clofibrate Impairs water excretion. Myositis.	40-70	15.0-17.5/30-110	92-97	0.14	500-1000 mg bid	I	q6-12h	q12-18h	Avoid	Hemo: None / CAPD: No data / CAVH: Dose for GFR 10-50
Colestipol Hyperchloremic acidosis.	None	Not absorbed	None	None	13-30 g q24h	D	100%	100%	100%	Hemo: None / CAPD: None / CAVH: Dose for GFR 10-50
Fluvastatin	< 1	0.5-1/No data	98	0.42	2-10 mg q24h	D	100%	100%	100%	Hemo: None / CAPD: No data / CAVH: Dose for GFR 10-50
Gemfibrozil	None	7.6/Unchanged	97-99	No data	600 mg bid	D	100%	100%	100%	Hemo: None / CAPD: No data / CAVH: Dose for GFR 10-50
Lovastatin	None	1.1-1.7/Unchanged	> 95	No data	20-80 mg q24h	D	100%	100%	100%	Hemo: No data / CAPD: No data / CAVH: Dose for GFR 10-50
Nicotinic acid Toxic reactions frequent in ESRD. Aspirin may attenuate flushing.	None	0.5-1/Unknown	No data	No data	1-2 g tid	D	100%	50%	25%	Hemo: No data / CAPD: No data / CAVH: Dose for GFR 10-50
Pravastatin	< 10	0.8-3.2/Unchanged	40-60	No data	10-40 mg q24h	D	100%	100%	100%	Hemo: No data / CAPD: No data / CAVH: Dose for GFR 10-50

For definitions of the abbreviations used in the tables, see page 16.

Miscellaneous Agents (Continued)

Drug, Toxicity Notes	Percent Excreted Unchanged	Half-Life (Normal/ ESRD)	Plasma Protein Binding	Volume of Distribution	Dose for Normal Renal Function	Adjustment for Renal Failure				Supplement for Dialysis
						Method	GFR, mL/min			
							>50	10-50	<10	
	%	h	%	L/kg						
Hypolipidemic Agents (Continued)										
Probucol	<2	23-47 d/No data	No data	No data	500 mg bid	D	100%	100%	100%	Hemo: No data CAPD: No data CAVH: Dose for GFR 10-50
Simvastatin	<0.5	2/No data	>95	No data	5-40 mg q24h	D	100%	100%	100%	Hemo: No data CAPD: No data CAVH: Dose for GFR 10-50
Miscellaneous Drugs (Various)										
Acetohydroxamic acid Substantial May accumulate in ESRD.		3.5-5.0/15-23	No data	No data	10-15 mg/kg q24h	D	100%	100%	Avoid	Hemo: No data CAPD: No data CAVH: No data
Cisapride	<5	7-10/Unchanged	98	2.4	5-10 mg tid	D	100%	100%	50%	Hemo: None CAPD: No data CAVH: 50-100%
Clodronate Hyperchloremic acidosis.	70-90	13/51	36	0.25	3-10 mg/kg	D	100%	25-50%	Avoid	Hemo: No data CAPD: No data CAVH: No data
Cyclosporine Nephrotoxic. Hypertension. Seizures and tremor. Inhibitors of hepatic metabolism may increase blood concentration.	<1	3-16/Unchanged	96-99	3.5-7.4	3-10 mg/kg q24h	D	100%	100%	100%	Hemo: None CAPD: None CAVH: 1

Drug				Dose	Method	GFR >50	GFR 10-50	GFR <10	Supplement
Desferoxamine	30-35	6/No data	No data	2.0-2.5	Acute: 1.0 g then 0.5 g q4-12h Chronic: 0.5-1.0 g q24h	D	100%	100%	100%	Hemo: No data CAPD: No data CAVH: Dose for GFR 10-50
Metoclopramide Extrapyramidal side effects increase in ESRD.	10-22	2.5-4.0/14-15	40	2-3.4	10-15 mg qid	D	100%	75%	50%	Hemo: None CAPD: No data CAVH: 50-75%
N-Acetylcysteine	30	2.3-6.0/No data	50	0.33-0.47	140 mg/kg load then 70 mg/kg q4h for 17 doses	D	100%	100%	75%	Hemo: No data CAPD: No data CAVH: 1
Ondansetron	<5	2.5-5.5/Unchanged	75	2	8-10 mg IV q6-12h	D	100%	100%	100%	Hemo: No data CAPD: No data CAVH: Dose for GFR 10-50
Pentoxifylline	None	0.8/Unchanged	None	2.4-4.2	400 mg tid	I	q8-12h	q12-24h	q24h	Hemo: No data CAPD: No data CAVH: 1

Neuromuscular Agents

Drug				Dose	Method	GFR >50	GFR 10-50	GFR <10	Supplement
Alcuronium	80-85	3.0-3.5/16	40	0.28-0.36	No data	D	100%	100%	Avoid	Hemo: No data CAPD: No data CAVH: Avoid
Alfentanil	<1	1.4-2.0/Unchanged	88-95	0.3-1.0	8-245 µg/kg load then 0.5-3 µg/kg/min	D	100%	100%	100%	Hemo: No data CAPD: No data CAVH: Dose for GFR 10-50
Atracurium	None	0.3-0.4/Unchanged	40-50	0.15-0.18	0.4-0.5 mg/kg load then 0.08-0.1 mg/kg q15-25min	D	100%	100%	100%	Hemo: No data CAPD: No data CAVH: None
Doxacurium	24-38	1.2-1.6/3.7	40	0.12-0.22	0.025-0.05 mg/kg	D	100%	50%	50%	Hemo: No data CAPD: No data CAVH: Dose for GFR 10-50

For definitions of the abbreviations used in the tables, see page 16.

Miscellaneous Agents (Continued)

Drug, Toxicity Notes	Percent Excreted Unchanged	Half-Life (Normal/ ESRD)	Plasma Protein Binding	Volume of Distribution	Dose for Normal Renal Function	Method	Adjustment for Renal Failure GFR, mL/min			Supplement for Dialysis
							>50	10-50	<10	
	%	h	%	L/kg						
Neuromuscular Agents (Continued)										
Etomidate	2	4-5/Unchanged	75	2.0-4.5	0.2-0.6 mg/kg	D	100%	100%	100%	Hemo: No data CAPD: No data CAVH: Dose for GFR 10-50
Fazadinium	40	1/Unchanged	17	0.18-0.23	1-2 mg/kg	D	100%	100%	100%	Hemo: No data CAPD: No data CAVH: Dose for GFR 10-50
Fentanyl	6-8	2.5-3.5/Unchanged	79-87	2-5	0.002-0.05 mg/kg	D	100%	100%	100%	Hemo: No data CAPD: No data CAVH: Dose for GFR 10-50
Gallamine Recurarization may occur up to 24 hours after dose. If blockade not responsive to neostigmine, dialysis may be useful.	85-100	2.3-2.7/6-20	30-70	0.21-0.24	0.5-1.5 mg/kg	D	75%	Avoid	Avoid	Hemo: Not applicable CAPD: Not applicable CAVH: Dose for GFR 10-50
Ketamine	2-3	2.0-3.5/Unchanged	No data	1.8-3.1	1.0-4.5 mg/kg	D	100%	100%	100%	Hemo: No data CAPD: No data CAVH: Dose for GFR 10-50
Metocurine	45-60	3.5-5.8/11.3	70	0.42-0.57	0.2-0.4 mg/kg	D	75%	50%	50%	Hemo: No data CAPD: No data CAVH: Dose for GFR 10-50
Mivacurium	No data	1.5-3.0	No data	0.1	4-10 µg/kg/min	D	100%	50%	50%	Hemo: No data CAPD: No data CAVH: No data

Drug	% Excreted Unchanged	Half-Life Normal/ESRD	Plasma Protein Binding (%)	Vd (L/kg)	Dose	Method	GFR >50	GFR 10-50	GFR <10	Adjustment for Dialysis
Neostigmine	67	1.3/3.0	None	0.5-1.0	15-375 mg q24h	D	100%	50%	25%	Hemo: No data CAPD: No data CAVH: Dose for GFR 10-50
Pancuronium Recurarization may occur up to 24 hours after dose.	30-40	1.7-2.2/4.3-8.2	70-85	0.15-0.38	0.04-0.1 mg/kg	D	100%	50%	Avoid	Hemo: No data CAPD: No data CAVH: Dose for GFR 10-50
Pipecuronium	38	2.3/4.4	No data	0.31	100 µg/kg	D	100%	50%	25%	Hemo: No data CAPD: No data CAVH: Dose for GFR 10-50
Propofol Green urine.	<0.3	1.5/16.8	96-99	8-19	2.0-2.5 mg/kg	D	100%	100%	100%	Hemo: No data CAPD: No data CAVH: Dose for GFR 10-50
Pyridostigmine Renal excretion decreased by basic drugs.	80-90	1.5-2.0/6	No data	0.8-1.4	60-1500 mg q24h	D	50%	35%	20%	Hemo: No data CAPD: No data CAVH: Dose for GFR 10-50
Succinylcholine Hyperkalemia in ESRD.	None	3/No data	No data	No data	0.3-1.1 mg/kg load then 0.04-0.07 mg/kg prn	D	100%	100%	100%	Hemo: No data CAPD: No data CAVH: Dose for GFR 10-50
Sufentanil	1-2	1-2/Unchanged	92	1.7-5.2	Anesthetic induction or 1-30 µg/kg	D	100%	100%	100%	Hemo: No data CAPD: No data CAVH: Dose for GFR 10-50
Tubocurarine Large or repetitive doses may result in prolonged effect. Recurarization may occur.	40-60	0.5-4/5.5	30-50	0.22-0.39	0.1-0.2 mg/kg	D	75%	50%	Avoid	Hemo: No data CAPD: No data CAVH: Dose for GFR 10-50
Vecuronium	25	0.5-1.3/Unchanged	30	0.18-0.27	0.08-0.1 mg/kg load then 0.01-0.05 mg/kg q12-15 min	D	100%	100%	100%	Hemo: No data CAPD: No data CAVH: Dose for GFR 10-50

For definitions of the abbreviations used in the tables, see page 16.

Miscellaneous Agents (Continued)

Drug, Toxicity Notes	Percent Excreted Unchanged	Half-Life (Normal/ ESRD)	Plasma Protein Binding	Volume of Distribution	Dose for Normal Renal Function	Adjustment for Renal Failure				Supplement for Dialysis
						Method	GFR, mL/min			
							>50	10-50	<10	
	%	h	%	L/kg						
Proton-Pump Inhibitors										
Lansoprazole	None	1.3-2.9/Unchanged	> 98	No data	15-60 mg q24h	D	100%	100%	100%	Hemo: No data CAPD: No data CAVH: No data
Omeprazole	Negligible	0.5-1/Unchanged	95	No data	20-60 mg q24h	D	100%	100%	100%	Hemo: No data CAPD: No data CAVH: No data

For definitions of the abbreviations used in the tables, see page 16.

Sedatives, Hypnotics, and Other Drugs Used in Psychiatry

Psychotherapeutic drugs are commonly given to patients with renal disease to relieve anxiety and depression. Excessive sedation is the most frequent adverse effect in patients with renal insufficiency. Because malaise, somnolence, and encephalopathy are also common uremic symptoms, recognition of the adverse drug reactions may be delayed.

Benzodiazepines are often used to treat emotional stress associated with decreasing renal function in patients on dialysis, although the efficacy of chronic benzodiazepine treatment has been questioned. Members of this class are generally safer than other antianxiety agents, and short-term administration is effective. Active polar metabolites of these compounds normally excreted by the kidneys are likely to accumulate in patients with renal impairment and produce enhanced, prolonged sedation. Diazepam, chlordiazepoxide, and flurazepam are examples of such compounds. Because of the potential for drug or metabolite accumulation, chronic use of these agents and others in this drug class should be discouraged in patients with decreased renal function.

Phenothiazines (which are used to treat major psychoses) and tricyclic antidepressants (which are used for severe depression in patients with renal disease) can also produce excessive sedation. Patients taking these drugs may also exhibit anticholinergic effects, orthostatic hypotension, confusion, and extrapyramidal symptoms.

Lithium carbonate has become an increasingly prescribed antidepressant. The drug is excreted by the kidney and has a narrow therapeutic range. Careful dose reduction and plasma lithium level monitoring are required in patients with impaired or unstable renal function. Hemodialysis has been used in cases of lithium overdose. Although lithium is effectively removed by dialysis, a rebound increase in plasma levels is common after hemodialysis, and repeated treatments may be required.

Sedatives, Hypnotics, and Other Drugs Used in Psychiatry

Drug, Toxicity Notes	Percent Excreted Unchanged	Half-Life (Normal/ESRD)	Plasma Protein Binding	Volume of Distribution	Dose for Normal Renal Function	Adjustment for Renal Failure — Method	Adjustment for Renal Failure — GFR, mL/min >50	Adjustment for Renal Failure — GFR, mL/min 10-50	Adjustment for Renal Failure — GFR, mL/min <10	Supplement for Dialysis
	%	h	%	L/kg						
Antidepressants										
Bupropion	Hepatic	10-21/No data	82-88	27-36	100 mg q8h	D	100%	100%	100%	Hemo: No data CAPD: No data CAVH: Not applicable
Nefazodone	Hepatic	2-4/Unchanged	99	0.22-0.87	100-600 mg q24h	D	100%	100%	100%	Hemo: No data CAPD: No data CAVH: Not applicable
Trazodone	Renal	6-11/No data	89-95	1-2	150-400 mg q24h	D	100%	No data	No data	Hemo: No data CAPD: No data CAVH: Not applicable
Venlafaxine	Hepatic	4/6-8	27	6-7	75-375 mg q24h	D	75%	50%	50%	Hemo: None CAPD: No data CAVH: Not applicable
Barbiturates										
Pentobarbital	Hepatic	18-48/Unchanged	60-70	1	30 mg q6-8h	D	100%	100%	100%	Hemo: None CAPD: No data CAVH: Dose for GFR 10-50

May cause excessive sedation, increase osteomalacia in ESRD. Charcoal hemoperfusion and hemodialysis more effective than peritoneal dialysis for poisoning.

						>50	10-50	<10	
Phenobarbital	Hepatic (renal)	60-150/117-160	40-60	0.7-1	50-100 mg q8-12h	I	q8-12h	q8-12h	q12-16h	Hemo: Dose after dialysis CAPD: 1/2 normal dose CAVH: Dose for GFR 10-50

Up to 50% unchanged drug excreted in urine with alkaline diuresis.

						>50	10-50	<10	
Secobarbital	Hepatic	20-35/No data	44	1.5-2.5	30-50 mg q6-8h	D	100%	100%	100%	Hemo: None CAPD: None CAVH: Not applicable
Thiopental	Hepatic	3.8/6-18	72-86	1.0-1.5	Anesthesia induction (individualized)	D	100%	100%	75%	Hemo: Not applicable CAPD: Not applicable CAVH: Not applicable

Benzodiazepines

May cause excessive sedation and encephalopathy in ESRD.

						>50	10-50	<10	
Alprazolam	Hepatic	9.5-19.0/Unchanged	70-80	0.9-1.3	0.25-5.0 mg q8h	D	100%	100%	100%	Hemo: None CAPD: No data CAVH: Not applicable
Chlordiazepoxide	Hepatic	5-30/Unchanged	94-97	0.3-0.5	15-100 mg q24h	D	100%	100%	50%	Hemo: None CAPD: No data CAVH: Dose for GFR 10-50
Clonazepam	Hepatic	18-50/No data	47	1.5-4.5	1.5 mg q24h	D	100%	100%	100%	Hemo: None CAPD: No data CAVH: Not applicable
Clorazepate	Hepatic (renal)	39-85/36	No data	1.3	15-60 mg q24h	D	100%	100%	100%	Hemo: No data CAPD: No data CAVH: Not applicable
Diazepam	Hepatic	20-90/Unchanged	94-98	0.7-3.4	5-40 mg q24h	D	100%	100%	100%	Hemo: None CAPD: No data CAVH: 1
Estazolam	Hepatic	8-24/No data	93	No data	1.0 mg qhs	D	100%	100%	100%	Hemo: No data CAPD: No data CAVH: Not applicable

For definitions of the abbreviations used in the tables, see page 16.

Sedatives, Hypnotics, and Other Drugs Used in Psychiatry (Continued)

Drug, Toxicity Notes	Percent Excreted Unchanged	Half-Life (Normal/ ESRD)	Plasma Protein Binding	Volume of Distribution	Dose for Normal Renal Function	Method	Adjustment for Renal Failure GFR, mL/min >50	10-50	<10	Supplement for Dialysis
	%	h	%	L/kg						
Benzodiazepines (Continued)										
Flurazepam	Hepatic	47-100/Unchanged	No data	3.4	15-30 mg qhs	D	100%	100%	100%	Hemo: None CAPD: No data CAVH: Not applicable
Lorazepam	Hepatic	5-10/32-70	87	0.9-1.3	1-2 mg q8-12h	D	100%	100%	100%	Hemo: None CAPD: No data CAVH: Dose for GFR 10-50
Midazolam	Hepatic	1.2-12.3/Unchanged	93-96	1.0-6.6	Individualized	D	100%	100%	50%	Hemo: Not applicable CAPD: Not applicable CAVH: Not applicable
Oxazepam	Hepatic	5-10/25-90	97	0.6-1.6	30-120 mg q24h	D	100%	100%	100%	Hemo: None CAPD: No data CAVH: Dose for GFR 10-50
Quazepam	Hepatic	20-40/No data	95	No data	15 mg qhs	D	No data	No data	No data	Hemo: Unknown CAPD: No data CAVH: Not applicable
Temazepam	Hepatic	4-10/No data	96	1.3-1.5	30 mg qhs	D	100%	100%	100%	Hemo: None CAPD: None CAVH: Not applicable
Triazolam	Hepatic	2-4/Unchanged	85-95	No data	0.25-0.50 mg qhs	D	100%	100%	100%	Hemo: None CAPD: None CAVH: Not applicable

Protein binding correlates with alpha-1 acid glycoprotein concentration.

Benzodiazepines: Benzodiazepine Antagonist

May cause excessive sedation and encephalopathy in ESRD.

Drug	Metabolism	Half-Life (Normal/ESRD)	Protein Binding	Vd	Dose	D/I	GFR >50	GFR 10-50	GFR <10	Supplement
Flumazenil	Hepatic	0.7-1.3/No data	40-50	0.6-1.1	0.2 mg IV over 15 sec	D	100%	100%	100%	Hemo: None / CAPD: No data / CAVH: Not applicable

Miscellaneous Sedative Agents

Drug	Metabolism	Half-Life (Normal/ESRD)	Protein Binding	Vd	Dose	D/I	GFR >50	GFR 10-50	GFR <10	Supplement
Buspirone	Hepatic	2-3/5.8	95	5	5.0 mg q8h	D	100%	100%	100%	Hemo: None / CAPD: No data / CAVH: Not applicable
Etchlorvynol	Hepatic	10-20/No data	35-50	10-20/No data	500 mg qhs	D	100%	Avoid	Avoid	Hemo: Avoid / CAPD: Avoid / CAVH: Not applicable
Haloperidol	Hepatic	10-19/No data	90-92	14-21	1-2 mg q8-12h	D	100%	100%	100%	Hemo: None / CAPD: None / CAVH: Dose for GFR 10-50
Lithium carbonate	Renal	14-28/40	None	0.5-0.9	0.9-1.2 g q24h	D	100%	50-75%	25-50%	Hemo: Dose after dialysis / CAPD: None / CAVH: Dose for GFR 10-50
Meprobamate	Hepatic (renal)	9-11/Unchanged	0-30	0.5-0.8	1.2-1.6 g q24h	I	q6h	q9-12h	q12-18h	Hemo: None / CAPD: No data / CAVH: Not applicable

Etchlorvynol: Removed by hemoperfusion. Excessive sedation.

Haloperidol: Hypotension, excessive sedation.

Lithium carbonate: Nephrotoxic. Nephrogenic diabetes insipidus. Nephrotic syndrome. Renal tubular acidosis. Interstitial fibrosis. Acute toxicity when serum levels > 1.2 mEq/L. Serum levels should be measured periodically 12 h after dose. $T_{1/2}$ does not reflect extensive tissue accumulation. Plasma levels rebound after dialysis. Toxicity enhanced by volume depletion, NSAIDs, and diuretics.

Meprobamate: Excessive sedation. Excretion enhanced by forced diuresis.

For definitions of the abbreviations used in the tables, see page 16.

Sedatives, Hypnotics, and Other Drugs Used in Psychiatry (Continued)

Drug, Toxicity Notes	Percent Excreted Unchanged	Half-Life (Normal/ ESRD)	Volume of Distribution	Plasma Protein Binding	Dose for Normal Renal Function	Adjustment for Renal Failure Method	GFR, mL/min >50	10-50	<10	Supplement for Dialysis
	%	h	L/kg	%						
Phenothiazines										
Orthostatic hypotension, extrapyramidal symptoms, and confusion can occur.										
Chlorpromazine	Hepatic	11-42/Unchanged	8-160	91-99	300-800 mg q24h	D	100%	100%	100%	Hemo: None CAPD: None CAVH: Dose for GFR 10-50
Promethazine Excessive sedation may occur in ESRD.	Hepatic	9-12/No data	Large	No data	20-100 mg q24h	D	100%	100%	100%	Hemo: No data CAPD: No data CAVH: Dose for GFR 10-50
Selective Serotonin-Reuptake Inhibitors (SSRIs)										
Fluoxetine $T_{1/2}$ of active metabolite is 7-9 days.	Hepatic	24-72/Unchanged	12-42	94.5	20 mg q24h	D	100%	100%	100%	Hemo: No data CAPD: No data CAVH: Not applicable
Fluvoxamine	Hepatic	12-15/Unchanged	25	77	100 mg q24h	D	100%	100%	100%	Hemo: None CAPD: No data CAVH: Not applicable
Paroxetine	Hepatic	10-16/30	13	95	20-60 mg q24h	D	100%	50-75%	0.5	Hemo: No data CAPD: No data CAVH: Not applicable
Sertraline	Hepatic	24/No data	25	97	50-200 mg q24h	D	100%	100%	100%	Hemo: No data CAPD: No data CAVH: Not applicable

Tricyclic Antidepressants

Anticholinergic side effects cause urinary retention and orthostatic hypotension. Drug may cause confusion and excessive sedation.

Drug		$T_{1/2}$ (Normal/ESRD)	%	Vd	Dose	Method	GFR >50	GFR 10-50	GFR <10	Supplement
Amitriptyline	Hepatic	24-40/Unchanged	96	6-36	25 mg q8h	D	100%	100%	100%	Hemo: None / CAPD: No data / CAVH: Not applicable
Amoxapine $T_{1/2}$ of active metabolite is 30 hours.	Hepatic	8-30/No data	90	No data	75-200 mg q24h	D	100%	100%	100%	Hemo: None / CAPD: No data / CAVH: Not applicable
Clomipramine	Hepatic	19-37/No data	97	No data	100-250 mg q24h	D	No data	No data	No data	Hemo: None / CAPD: No data / CAVH: Not applicable
Desipramine	Hepatic	18-26/No data	92	10-50	100-200 mg q24h	D	100%	100%	100%	Hemo: None / CAPD: None / CAVH: Not applicable
Doxepin	Hepatic	8-25/10-30	95	9-33	25 mg q8h	D	100%	100%	100%	Hemo: None / CAPD: None / CAVH: Dose for GFR 10-50
Imipramine	Hepatic	12-24/No data	96	10-20	25 mg q8h	D	100%	100%	100%	Hemo: None / CAPD: None / CAVH: Not applicable
Nortriptyline	Hepatic	25-38/15-66	95	15-23	25 mg q6-8h	D	100%	100%	100%	Hemo: None / CAPD: None / CAVH: Not applicable
Protryptyline	Hepatic	54-98/No data	92	15-31	15-60 mg q24h	D	100%	100%	100%	Hemo: None / CAPD: None / CAVH: Not applicable
Trimipramine	Hepatic	24/No data	90-96	31	50-150 mg q24h	D	100%	100%	100%	Hemo: None / CAPD: None / CAVH: Not applicable

For definitions of the abbreviations used in the tables, see page 16.

Bibliography

Analgesics

NARCOTICS AND NARCOTIC ANTAGONISTS

Alfentanil

Chauvin M, Lebrault C, Levron JC, et al. Pharmacokinetics of alfentanil in chronic renal failure. Anesth Analg. 1987;66:53-6.

Mather LE. Opioid pharmacokinetics in relation to their effects [Review]. Anaesth Intensive Care. 1987;66:13-6.

Meistelman C, Saint-Maurice C, Lepaul M, et al. A comparison of alfentanil pharmacokinetics in children and adults. Anesthesiology. 1987;66:13-6.

Persson MP, Nilsson A, Hartvig P. Pharmacokinetics of alfentanil in total I.V. anaesthesia. Br J Anaesth. 1988;60:755-61.

Scholz J, Steinfath M, Scholz M. Clinical pharmacokinetics of alfentanil, fentanyl and sufentanil. An update. Clin Pharmacokinet. 1996;31:275-92.

Sitar DS, Duke PC, Benthuysen JL, et al. Aging and alfentanil disposition in healthy volunteers and surgical patients. Can J Anaesth. 1989;36:149-54.

Butorphanol

Gillis C, Benfield P, Goa KL. Transnasal butorphanol. Drugs. 1995;50:157-175.

Ramsey R, Higbee M, Maesner J, et al. Influence of age on the pharmacokinetics of butorphanol. Pharmacol Toxicol. 1987;60(Suppl 2):8-16.

Codeine

Davies G, Kingswood C, Street M. Pharmacokinetics of opiods in renal dysfunction. Clin Pharmacokinet. 1996;31:410-22.

Elseviers MM, DeBroe ME. Combination analgesic involvement in the pathogenesis of analgesic nephropathy. The European prospective. Am J Kid Dis. 1996;28(Suppl 1):S48-S55.

Quiding H, Anderson P, Bondesson U, et al. Plasma concentrations of codeine and its metabolite, morphine, after single and repeated oral administration. Eur J Clin Pharmacol. 1986;30:673-7.

99

Fentanyl

Cleary JF. Pharmacokinetic and pharmacodynamic issues in the treatment of break-through pain. Semin Oncol. 1997;24(Suppl 16):S16-9.

Davies G, Kingswood C, Street M. Pharmacokinetics of opiods in renal dysfunction. Clin Pharmacokinet. 1996;31:410-22.

Reilly CS, Wood AJ, Wood M. Variability of fentanyl pharmacokinetics in man: computer predicted plasma concentrations for three intravenous dosage regimens. Anaesthesia. 1985;40:837-43.

Wagner BK, O'Hara DA. Pharmacokinetics and pharmacodynamics of sedatives and analgesics in the treatment of agitated critically ill patients. Clin Pharmacokinet. 1997;33:426-53.

Meperidine

Claric RF, Wei EM, Anderson PO. Meperidine: therapeutic use and toxicity. J Emer Med. 1995;13:797-802.

Davies G, Kingswood C, Street M. Pharmacokinetics of opiods in renal dysfunction. Clin Pharmacokinet. 1996;31:410-22.

Sjöström S, Hartvig P, Persson MP, et al. Pharmacokinetics of epidural morphine and meperidine in humans. Anesthesiology. 1987;67:877-88.

Sjöström S, Tamsen A, Persson MP, et al. Pharmacokinetics of intrathecal morphine and meperidine in humans. Anesthesiology. 1987;667:889-95.

Methadone

Bertschy G. Methadone maintenance treatment: an update. Eur Arch Psychiatry Clin Neurosci. 1995;245:114-24.

Inturrisi CE, Colburn WA, Kaiko RF, et al. Pharmacokinetics and pharmacodynamics of methadone in patients with chronic pain. Clin Pharmacol Ther. 1987;41:392-401.

Quinn DI, Wodak A, Day RO. Pharmacokinetic and pharmacodynamic principles of illicit drug use and treatment of illicit drug users. Clin Pharmacokinet. 1997;33:344-400.

Sawe J. High-dose morphine and methadone in cancer patients: clinical pharmacokinetic considerations of oral treatment [Review]. Clin Pharmacokinet. 1986;11:87-106.

Morphine

Benyhe S. Morphine: new aspects in the study of an ancient compound [Review]. Life Sci. 1994;55:969-79.

Chauvin M, Sandouk P, Scherrmann JM, et al. Morphine pharmacokinetics in renal failure. Anesthesiology. 1987;66:327-31.

Davies G, Kingswood C, Street M. Pharmacokinetics of opiods in renal dysfunction. Clin Pharmacokinet. 1996;31:410-22.

Rushton AR, Sneyd JR. Opioid analgesics. Br J Hosp Med. 1997;57:105-6.

Sawe J. High-dose morphine and methadone in cancer patients. Clinical pharmacokinetic considerations of oral treatment [Review]. Clin Pharmacokinet. 1986;11:87-106.

Sjostrom S, Hartvig P, Persson MP, et al. Pharmacokinetics of epidural morphine and meperidine in humans. Anesthesiology. 1987;667:877-88.

Upton RN, Semple TJ, Macintyre PE. Pharmacokinetic optimization of opioid treatment in acute pain therapy. Clin Pharmacokinet. 1997;33:225-44.

Wagner BK, O'Hara DA. Pharmacokinetics and pharmacodynamics of sedatives and analgesics in the treatment of agitated critically ill patients. Clin Pharmacokinet. 1997;33:426-53.

Naloxone

Bowden CA, Krenzelok EP. Clinical applications of commonly used contemporary antidotes. Drug Safety. 1997;16:9-47.

Cherny NI. Opiod analgesics: comparative features and prescribing guidelines. Drugs. 1996;51:713-37.

Pentazocine

Forcyki Z, Martens F, Thalhofer S, et al. Tranquilizers, analgesics and antidepressants in patients treated with hemodialysis [Review]. Blood Purif. 1985;3:109-19.

Mather LE. Opioid pharmacokinetics in relation to their effects. Anaesth Intensive Care. 1987;15:15-22.

Yeh SY, Todd GD, Johnson RE, et al. The pharmacokinetics of pentazocine and tripelannamine. Clin Pharmacol Ther. 1986;39:669-76.

Propoxyphene

Colburn WA, Inturrisi CE. Propoxyphene: accumulation or altered kinetics? [Letter]. Eur J Clin Pharmacol. 1985;28:725-6.

Sufentanil

Davis PJ, Stiller RL, Cook DR, et al. Pharmacokinetics of sufentanil in adolescent patients with chronic renal failure. Anesth Analg. 1988;67:268-71.

Fyman PN, Reynolds JR, Moser F, et al. Pharmacokinetics of sufentanil in patients undergoing renal transplantation. Can Anaesth. 1988;35:312-5.

Wiggum DC, Cork RC, Weldon ST, et al. Postoperative respiratory depression and elevated sufentanil levels in a patient with chronic renal failure. Anesthesiology. 1985;63:708-10.

NON-NARCOTICS

Acetaminophen

Blantz RC. Acetaminophen: acute and chronic effects on renal failure. Am J Kid Dis. 1996;28(Suppl 1):S3-6.

Clissold SP. Paracetamol and phenacetin. Drugs. 1986;32(Suppl 4):46-59.

D'Arcy PF. Paracetamol. Adverse Drug React Toxicol Rev. 1997;16:9-14.

Segasothy M, Suleiman AB, Puvaneswary M, et al. Paracetamol: a cause for analgesic nephropathy and end-stage renal disease. Nephron. 1988;50:50-4.

Aspirin (USP)

Clissold SP. Aspirin and related derivatives of salicylic acid. Drugs. 1986;32(Suppl 4):8-26.

Montgomery PR, Berger LG, Mitenko PA, et al. Salicylate metabolism: effects of age and sex in adults. Clin Pharmacol Ther. 1986;39:571-6.

Montgomery PR, Sitar DS. Acetylsalicylic acid metabolites in blood and urine after plain- and enteric-coated tablets. Biopharm Drug Dispos. 1986;7:21-5.

Needs CJ, Brooks PM. Clinical pharmacokinetics of the salicylates. Clin Pharmacokinet. 1985;10:165-77.

Antihypertensive and Cardiovascular Agents

ANTIHYPERTENSIVE DRUGS

ADRENERGIC AND SEROTONINERGIC MODULATORS

Clonidine

Langley MS, Heel RC. Transdermal clonidine: a preliminary review of its pharmacodynamic properties and therapeutic efficacy. Drugs. 1988;35:123-42.

Lowenthal DT, Matzek KM, MacGregor TR. Clinical pharmacokinetics of clonidine. Clin Pharmacokinet. 1988;14:287-310.

Doxazosin

Carlson RV, Bailey RR, Begg EJ, et al. Pharmacokinetics and effect on blood pressure of doxazosin in normal subjects and patients with renal failure. Clin Pharmacol Ther. 1986;40:561-6.

Oliver RM, Upward JW, Dewhurst AG, et al. The pharmacokinetics of doxazosin in patients with hypertension and renal impairment. Br J Clin Pharm. 1990;29:417-22.

Fulton B, Wagstaff AJ, Sorkin EM. Doxazosin: an update of its clinical pharmacology and therapeutic application in hypertension and benign prostatic hypertrophy. Drugs. 1995;49:295-320.

Guanabenz

Gehr M, McCarthy EP, Goldberg M. Guanabenz: a centrally acting, natriuretic antihypertensive drug. Kidney Int. 1986;29:1203-8.

Holmes B, Brogden RN, Heel RC, et al. Guanabenz: a review of its pharmacodynamic properties and therapeutic efficacy in hypertension. Drugs. 1983;26:212-29.

Guanadrel

Finnerty FA, Brogden RN. Guanadrel: a review of its pharmacodynamics and pharmacokinetic properties and therapeutic use in hypertension. Drugs. 1985;30:22-31.

Halstenson CE, Opsahl JA, Abraham PA, et al. Disposition of guanadrel in subjects with normal and impaired renal function. J Clin Pharmacol. 1989;29:128-32.

Guanethidine

No references

Guanfacine

Carchman SH, Sica DA, Davis J, et al. Steady-state plasma levels and pharmacokinetics of guanfacine in patients with renal insufficiency. Nephron. 1989;53:18-23.

Sorkin EM, Heel RC. Guanfacine: a review of its pharmacodynamic and pharmacokinetic properties, and therapeutic efficacy in the treatment of hypertension. Drugs. 1986;31:301-36.

Ketanserin

Ebihara A, Fugimura A. Metabolites of antihypertensive drugs. Clin Pharmacokinet. 1991;21:331-43.

Persson B, Heykants J, Hedner T. Clinical pharmacokinetics of ketanserin. Clin Pharmacokinet. 1991;20:263-79.

Methyldopa

Myhre E, Rugstad HE, Hansen T. Clinical pharmacokinetics of methyldopa. Clin Pharmacokinet. 1982;7:221-33.

Prazosin

Lameire N, Gordts J. A pharmacokinetic study of prazosin in patients with varying degrees of chronic renal failure. Eur J Clin Pharmacol. 1986;31:333-7.

Vincent J, Meredith PA, Reid JL, et al. Clinical pharmacokinetics of prazosin. Clin Pharmacokinet. 1985;10:144-54.

Reserpine

Zsoter TT, Johnson GE, Deveber GA, et al. Excretion and metabolism of reserpine in renal failure. Clin Pharmacol Ther. 1973;14:325-30.

Terazosin

Achari R, Laddu A. Terazosin: a new alpha-adrenoreceptor blocking drug. J Clin Pharmacol. 1992;32:520-3.

Titmarsh S, Monk JP. Terazosin: a review of its pharmacodynamic and pharmacokinetic properties, and therapeutic efficacy in essential hypertension. Drugs. 1987;33:461-77.

ANGIOTENSIN-II–RECEPTOR ANTAGONISTS

Losartan

Goa KL, Wagstaff AJ. Losartan potassium: a review of its pharmacology, clinical efficacy and tolerability in the management of hypertension. Drugs. 1996;51:820-45.

Sica DA, Lo MW, Shaw WC, et al. The pharmacokinetics of losartan in renal insufficiency. J Hypertens. 1995;13:S49-S52.

ANGIOTENSIN-CONVERTING–ENZYME INHIBITORS

Benazepril

Balfour JA, Goa KL. Benazepril: a review of its pharmacodynamic and pharmacokinetic properties and therapeutic efficacy in hypertension and congestive heart failure. Drugs. 1991;42:511-39.

Captopril

Brogden RN, Todd PA, Sorkin EM. Captopril: an update of its pharmacodynamic and pharmacokinetic properties, and therapeutic use in hypertension and congestive heart failure. Drugs. 1988;36:540-600.

Fujimura A, Kajiyama H, Ebihara A, et al. Pharmacokinetics and pharmacodynamics of captopril in patients undergoing continuous ambulatory peritoneal dialysis. Nephron. 1986;44:324-8.

Cilazapril

Deget F, Brogden RN. Cilazapril: a review of its pharmacodynamic and pharmacokinetic properties, and therapeutic potential in cardiovascular disease. Drugs. 1991;41:799-820.

Kloke HJ, Ambros RJ, Van Hamersvelt HW, et al. Pharmacokinetics and haemodynamic effects of the angiotensin-converting enzyme inhibitor cilazapril in hypertensive patients with normal and impaired renal function. Br J Clin Pharmacol. 1996;42:615-20.

Enalapril

Mujais S, Quintanilla A, Zahid M, et al. Renal handling of enalaprilat. Am J Kid Dis. 1992;19:121-5.

Todd PA, Goa KL. Enalapril: a reappraisal of its pharmacology and therapeutic use in hypertension. Drugs. 1992;43:346-61.

Fosinopril

Gehr T, Sica D, Grasela D, et al. Fosinopril pharmacokinetics and pharmacodynamics in chronic ambulatory peritoneal dialysis patients. Eur J Clin Pharmacol. 1991;41:165-9.

Wagstaff AJ, Davis R, McTavish D. Fosinopril: a reappraisal of its pharmacology and therapeutic efficacy in essential hypertension. Drugs. 1996;51:777-91.

Lisinopril

Lancaster SG, Todd PA. Lisinopril: a preliminary review of its pharmacodynamic and pharmacokinetic properties, and therapeutic use in hypertension and congestive heart failure. Drugs. 1988;35:646-9.

Neubeck M, Fliser D, Pritsch M, et al. Pharmacokinetics and pharmacodynamics of lisinopril in advanced renal failure. Eur J Clin Pharmacol. 1994;46:537-43.

Pentopril

Rakhit A, Radensky P, Szerlip HM, et al. Effect of renal impairment on disposition of pentopril and its active metabolite. Clin Pharmacol Ther. 1988;44:39-48.

Perindopril

Guerin A, Resplandy G, Marchais S, et al. The effect of haemodialysis on the pharmacokinetics of perindoprilat after long-term perindopril. Eur J Clin Pharmacol. 1993;44:183-87.

Sennesael J, Ali A, Sweny P, et al. The pharmacokinetics of perindopril and its effects on serum angiotensin-converting enzyme activity in hypertensive patients with chronic renal failure. Br J Clin Pharmac. 1992;33:93-9.

Quinapril

Halstenson CE, Opsahl JA, Rachael K, et al. The pharmacokinetics of quinapril and its active metabolite quinaprilat in patients with varying degrees of renal function. J Clin Pharmacol. 1992;32:344-50.

Plosker GL, Sorkin EM. Quinapril: a reappraisal of its pharmacology and therapeutic efficacy in cardiovascular disorders. Drugs. 1994;48:227-52.

Wolter K, Fritschka E. Pharmacokinetics and pharmacodynamics of quinaprilat after low dose quinapril in patients with terminal renal failure. Eur J Clin Pharmacol. 1993;44:S53-6.

Ramipril

Fillastre JP, Baguet JC, Dubois D, et al. Kinetics, safety, and efficacy of ramipril after long-term administration in hemodialyzed patients. J Cardiovasc Pharmacol. 1996;27:269-74.

Frampton JE, Peters DH. Ramipril: an updated review of its therapeutic use in essential hypertension and heart failure. Drugs. 1995;49:440-66.

Meisel S, Shamiss A, Rosenthal T. Clinical pharmacokinetics of ramipril. Clin Pharmacokinet. 1994;26:7-15.

BETA-BLOCKERS

Acebutolol

Singh BN, Thoden WR, Ward A. Acebutolol: a review of its pharmacological properties and therapeutic efficacy in hypertension, angina pectoris and arrhythmia. Drugs. 1985;29:531-69.

Atenolol

Wadworth AN, Murdoch D, Brogden RN. Atenolol: a reappraisal of its pharmacological properties and therapeutic use in cardiovascular disorders. Drugs. 1991;41;468-510.

Betaxolol

Frishman WH, Tepper D, Lazar EJ, et al. Betaxolol: a new long-acting beta-1 selective adrenergic blocker. J Clin Pharmacol. 1990;30:686-92.

Bisoprolol

Johns TE, Lopez LM. Bisoprolol: is this just another beta-blocker for hypertension or angina? Ann Pharmacother. 1995;29:403-14.

Lancaster SG, Sorkin EM. Bisoprolol: a preliminary review of its pharmacodynamic and pharmacokinetic properties, and therapeutic efficacy in hypertension and angina pectoris. Drugs. 1988;36:256-85.

Bopindolol

Harron D, Goa KL, Langtry H. Bopindolol: a review of its pharmacodynamic and pharmacokinetic properties and therapeutic efficacy. Drugs. 1991;41:130-49.

Carteolol

Amemiya M, Tabei K, Furuya H, et al. Pharmacokinetics of carteolol in patients with impaired renal function. Eur J Clin Pharmacol. 1992;43:417-21.

Hasenfub G, Schafer-Korting M, Knauf H, et al. Pharmacokinetics of carteolol in relation to renal function. Eur J Clin Pharmacol. 1985;29:461-5.

Carvedilol

McTavish D, Campoli-Richards D, Sorkin EM. Carvedilol: a review of its pharmacodynamic and pharmacokinetic properties, and therapeutic efficacy. Drugs. 1993;45:232-58.

Morgan T. Clinical pharmacokinetics and pharmacodynamics of carvedilol. Clin Pharmacokinet. 1994;26:335-46.

Celiprolol

Milne RJ, Buckley M. Celiprolol: an updated review of its pharmacodynamic and pharmacokinetic properties, and therapeutic efficacy in cardiovascular disease. Drugs. 1991;41:941-69.

Dilevalol

Chrisp P, Goa KL. Dilevalol: a review of its pharmacodynamic and pharmacokinetic properties and therapeutic potential in hypertension. Drugs. 1990;39:234-63.

Kelly JG, Laher MS, Donohue J, et al. The pharmacokinetics of dilevalol in renal impairment. J Human Hypertens. 1990;4:59-62.

Esmolol

Wiest D. Esmolol: a review of its therapeutic efficacy and pharmacokinetic characteristics. Clin Pharmacokinet. 1995;28:190-02.

Labetalol

Goa KL, Benfield P, Sorkin EM. Labetalol: a reappraisal of its pharmacology, pharmacokinetic properties and therapeutic use in hypertension and ischaemic heart disease. Drugs. 1989;37:538-27.

Halstenson CE, Opsahl JA, Pence TV, et al. The disposition and dynamics of labetalol in patients on dialysis. Clin Pharmacol Ther. 1986;40:462-8.

Metoprolol

Regardh CG, Johnsson G. Clinical pharmacokinetics of metoprolol. Clin Pharmacokinet. 1980;5:557-69.

Nadolol

Frishman WH. Nadolol: a new beta-adrenoceptor antagonist. N Engl J Med. 1981;305:678-82.

Penbutolol

Bernard N, Cuisinaud G, Pozet N, et al. Pharmacokinetics of penbutolol and its metabolites in renal insufficiency. Eur J Clin Pharmacol. 1985;29:215-9.
Sclanz KD, Thomas RL. Penbutolol: a new beta-adrenergic blocking agent. Ann Pharmacother. 1990;24:403-8.

Pindolol

Ohnhaus EE, Heidemann H, Meier J, et al. Metabolism of pindolol in patients with renal failure. Eur J Clin Pharmacol. 1982;22:423-8.

Propranolol

Stone WJ, Walle T. Massive propranolol metabolite retention during maintenance hemodialysis. Clin Pharmacol Ther. 1980;28:449-55.
Wood AJ, Vestal RE, Spannuth CL, et al. Propranolol disposition in renal failure. Br J Clin Pharmacol. 1980;10:561-6.

Sotalol

Fitton A, Sorkin EM. Sotalol: an updated review of its pharmacological properties and therapeutic use in cardiac arrhythmias. Drugs. 1993;46:678-719.

Timolol

Sproat TT, Lopez LM. Around the beta-blockers, one more time. Ann Pharmacother. 1991;25:962-71.

VASODILATORS

Diazoxide

Pearson RM. Pharmacokinetics and response to diazoxide in renal failure. Clin Pharmacokinet. 1977;2:198-204.

Hydralazine

Ludden TM, McNay JL, Shephard AM, et al. Clinical pharmacokinetics of hydralazine. Clin Pharmacokinet. 1982;7:185-205.

Reece PA. Hydralazine and related compounds: chemistry, metabolism, and mode of action. Med Res Rev. 1981;1:73-96.

Minoxidil

Halstenson CE, Opsahl JA, Wright E, et al. Disposition of minoxidil in patients with various degrees of renal function. J Clin Pharmacol. 1989;29:798-802.

Nitroprusside

Rindone JP, Sloane EP. Cyanide toxicity from sodium nitroprusside: risks and management. Ann Pharmacother. 1992;26:515-20.

Schulz V. Clinical pharmacokinetics of nitroprusside, cyanide, thiosulfate and thiocyanate. Clin Pharmacokinet. 1984;9:239-51.

CARDIOVASCULAR AGENTS

ANTIARRHYTHMIC AGENTS

N-*Acetylprocainamide*

Connolly SJ, Kates RE. Clinical pharmacokinetics of N-acetylprocainamide. Clin Pharmacokinet. 1982;7:205-20.

Domoto DT, Brown WW, Bruggensmith P. Removal of toxic levels of N-acetylprocainamide with continuous arteriovenous hemodiafiltration. Ann Intern Med. 1987;106:550-2.

Vlasses PH, Ferguson RK, Rocci ML Jr, et al. Lethal accumulation of procainamide metabolite in severe renal insufficiency. Am J Nephrol. 1986;6:112-6.

Adenosine

Faulds D, Chrisp P, Buckley MMT. Adenosine: an evaluation of its use in cardiac diagnostic procedures, and in the treatment of paroxysmal supraventricular tachycardia. Drugs. 1991;41:596-624.

Amiodarone

Gill J, Heel RC, Fitton A. Amiodarone: an overview of its pharmacological properties and review of its therapeutic use in cardiac arrhythmias. Drugs. 1992;43:69-110.

Mamprin F, Mullins P, Graham T, et al. Amiodarone-cyclosporine interaction in cardiac transplantation. Am Heart J. 1991;123:1725-6.

Roden DM. Pharmacokinetics of amiodarone: implications for drug therapy. Am J Cardiol. 1993;72:45F-50F.

Ujhelyi MR, Klamerus KJ, Vadiei K, et al. Disposition of intravenous amiodarone in subjects with normal and impaired renal function. J Clin Pharmacol. 1996;36:122-30.

Bretylium

Adir J, Narang PK, Josselson J. Nomogram for bretylium dosing in renal impairment. Ther Drug Monit. 1985;7:265-8.

Josselson J, Narang PK, Adir J, et al. Bretylium kinetics in renal insufficiency. Clin Pharmacol Ther. 1983;33:144-50.

Rappeport WG. Clinical pharmacokinetics of bretylium. Clin Pharmacokinet. 1985;10:248-56.

Cibenzoline

Aronoff G, Brier M, Mayer ML, et al. Bioavailability and kinetics of cibenzoline in patients with normal and impaired renal function. J Clin Pharmacol. 1991;31:38-44.

Harron DW, Brogden RN, Faulds D, et al. Cibenzoline: a review of its pharmacological properties and therapeutic potential in arrhythmias. Drugs. 1992;43:734-59.

Massarella JW, Khoo KC, Aogaichi K, et al. Effect of renal impairment on the pharmacokinetics of cibenzoline. Clin Pharmacol Ther. 1988;43:317-23.

Disopyramide

Brogden RN, Todd PA. Disopyramide: a reappraisal of its pharmacodynamic and pharmacokinetic properties, and therapeutic use in cardiac arrhythmias. Drugs. 1987;34:151-87.

Siddoway LA, Woosley RL. Clinical pharmacokinetics of disopyramide. Clin Pharmacokinet. 1986;11:214-22.

Flecainide

Forland SC, Burgess E, Blair AD, et al. Oral flecainide pharmacokinetics in patients with impaired renal function. J Clin Pharmacol. 1988;28:259-67.

William AJ, McQuinn RL, Walls J. Pharmacokinetics of flecainide acetate in patients with severe renal impairment. Clin Pharmacol Ther. 1988;43:449-55.

Lidocaine

Bennett PN, Aarons LJ, Bending MR, et al. Pharmacokinetics of lidocaine and its de-ethylated metabolite: dose and time dependency studies in man. J Pharmacokinet Biopharm. 1982;10:265-81.

Mexiletine

Campbell RW. Mexiletine. N Engl J Med. 1987;316:29-34.

Evers J, Messer W, Aboudan F, et al. Mexiletin Beiterminaler Nierenin-Suffizienz und Verschiedenen dialysererfahren. Klin Wochenschr. 1989;67:995-8.

Wang T, Wuellner D, Woosley RL, et al. Pharmacokinetics and non-dialyzability of mexiletine in renal failure. Clin Pharmacol Ther. 1985;37:649-53.

Moricizine

Pieniaszek HJ Jr, McEntegart CM, Mayersohn M, et al. Moricizine pharmacokinetics in renal insufficiency: reevaluation of elimination half-life. J Clin Pharmacol. 1992;32:412-4.

Procainamide

Bauer LA, Black D, Gensler A, et al. Influence of age, renal function and heart failure on procainamide clearance and N-acetylprocainamide serum concentrations. J Clin Pharmacol Ther Toxicol. 1989;27:213-6.

Raehl CL, Moorthy AV, Beirne GJ. Procainamide pharmacokinetics in patients on continuous ambulatory peritoneal dialysis. Nephron. 1986;44:191-4.

Propafenone

Bryson HM, Palmer KJ, Langtry HD, et al. Propafenone: a reappraisal of its pharmacology, pharmacokinetics and therapeutic use in cardiac arrhythmias. Drugs. 1993;45:85-130.

Fromm MF, Botsch S, Heinkele G, et al. Influence of renal function on the steady-state pharmacokinetics of the antiarrhythmic drug propafenone and its Phase I and Phase II metabolites. Eur J Clin Pharmacol. 1995;48:279-83.

Parker RB, McCollam PL, Bauman JL. Propafenone: a novel type Ic antiarrhythmic agent. Drug Intell Clin Pharm. 1989;23:196-203.

Quinidine

Kessler KM, Perez GO. Decreased quinidine plasma protein binding during hemodialysis. Clin Pharmacokinet. 1981;30:121-6.

Ochs HR, Greenblatt DJ, Woo E. Clinical pharmacokinetics of quinidine. Clin Pharmacokinet. 1980;5:150-68.

Tocainide

Braun J, Sorgel F, Engelmaier F, et al. Pharmacokinetics of tocainide in patients with severe renal failure. Eur J Clin Pharmacol. 1985;28:665-70.

Raehl CL, Beirne GJ, Moorthy AV, et al. Tocainide pharmacokinetics during continuous ambulatory peritoneal dialysis. Am J Cardiol. 1987;60:747-50.

Roden DM, Woosley RL. Tocainide. N Engl J Med. 1986;315:41-5.

CALCIUM-CHANNEL BLOCKERS

Amlodipine

Haria M, Wagstaff AJ. Amlodipine: a reappraisal of its pharmacological properties and therapeutic use in cardiovascular disease. Drugs. 1995;50:560-86.

Bepridil

Hollingshead LM, Faulds D, Fitton A. Bepridil: a review of its pharmacological properties and therapeutic use in stable angina pectoris. Drugs. 1992;44:835-57.

Diltiazem

Buckley MMT, Grant SM, Goa KL, et al. Diltiazem: a reappraisal of its pharmacological properties and therapeutic use. Drugs. 1990;39:757-806.

Patel R, Lipper B, Schwartzbard A, et al. Toxic effects of diltiazem in a patient with chronic renal failure. J Clin Pharmacol 1994;34:273-4.

Felodipine

Burr T, Larsson R, Regardh C, et al. Pharmacokinetics of felodipine in chronic hemodialysis patients. J Clin Pharmacokinet. 1991;31:709-13.

Todd PA, Faulds D. Felodipine: a review of its pharmacology and therapeutic use of the extended-release formulation in cardiovascular disorders. Drugs. 1992;44:251-77.

Isradipine

Brogden RN, Sorkin EM. Isradipine: an update of its pharmacodynamic and pharmacokinetic properties and therapeutic efficacy in the treatment of mild to moderate hypertension. Drugs. 1995;49:618-49.

Chandler MH, Schran HF, Cutler RE, et al. The effects of renal function on the disposition of isradipine. J Clin Pharmacol. 1988;28:1076-80.

Fitton A, Benfield P. Isradipine: a review of its pharmacodynamic and pharmacokinetic properties and therapeutic use in cardiovascular disease. Drugs. 1990;40:31-74.

Nicardipine

Ahmed JH, Grant AC, Rodgers RS, et al. Inhibitory effect of uremia on hepatic clearance and metabolism of nicardipine. J Clin Pharmacol. 1991;32:57-62.

Sorkin EM, Clissold SP. Nicardipine: a review of its pharmacodynamic and pharmacokinetic properties, and therapeutic efficacy, in the treatment of angina pectoris, hypertension and related cardiovascular disorders. Drugs. 1987;33:296-345.

Nifedipine

Grundy JS, Foster RT. The nifedipine gastrointestinal therapeutic system (GITS): evaluation of pharmaceutical, pharmacokinetic and pharmacological properties. Clin Pharmacokinet. 1996;30:28-51.

Kleinbloesem CH, Van Brummelen P, Woittiez AJ, et al. Influence of haemodialysis on the pharmacokinetics and haemodynamic effects of nifedipine during continuous intravenous infusion. Clin Pharmacokinet. 1986;11:316-22.

Sorkin EM, Clissold SP, Brogden RN. Nifedipine: a review of its pharmacodynamic and pharmacokinetic properties and therapeutic efficacy, in ischaemic heart disease, hypertension and related cardiovascular disorders. Drugs. 1985;30:182-274.

Nimodipine

Langley MS, Sorkin EM. Nimodipine: a review of its pharmacodynamic and pharmacokinetic properties, and therapeutic potential in cerebrovascular disease. Drugs. 1989;37:669-99.

Nisoldipine

Mitchell J, Frishman W, Heiman M. Nisoldipine: a new dihydropyridine calcium-channel blocker. J Clin Pharmacol. 1993;33:46-52.

Shionoiri H, Minamisawa K, Masumori S, et al. Pharmacokinetics and pharmacodynamics of nisoldipine in hypertensive patients with normal and mild to moderate impaired renal function. Drug Res. 1995;45:785-89.

Verapamil

Brogden RN, Benfield P. Verapamil: a review of its pharmacological properties and therapeutic use in coronary artery disease. Drugs. 1996;51:792-819.

Pritza DR, Bierman MH, Hammeke MD. Acute toxic effects of sustained release verapamil in chronic renal failure. Arch Intern Med. 1991;151:2081-4.

CARDIAC GLYCOSIDES

Digitoxin

Kelly RA, Smith TW. Use and misuse of digitalis blood levels. Heart Dis Stroke. 1992;1:117-22.

Vohringer HF, Rietbrock N. Digitalis therapy in renal failure with special regard to digitoxin. Int J Clin Pharmacol Res. 1981;19:175-84.

Digoxin

Sonnenblick M, Abraham AS, Meshulam Z, et al. Correlation between manifestations of digoxin toxicity and serum digoxin, calcium, potassium, and magnesium concentrations and arterial pH. BMJ. 1983;286:1089-91.

Ouabain

Ochs HR, Greenblatt DJ, Bodem G. Disease-related alterations in cardiac glycoside disposition. Clin Pharmacokinet. 1982;7:434-51.

DIURETICS

Acetazolamide

Chapron DJ, Gomolin IH, Sweeney KR. Acetazolamide blood concentrations are excessive in the elderly: propensity for acidosis and relationship to renal function. J Clin Pharmacol. 1989;29:348-53.

Roy LF, Dufresne LR, Legault L, et al. Acetazolamide in hemodialysis patients: a rational use after ocular surgery. Am J Kidney Dis. 1992;20:650-2.

Schwenk MH, St. Peter WL, Meese MG, et al. Acetazolamide toxicity and pharmacokinetics in patients receiving hemodialysis. Pharmacotherapy. 1995;15:522-7.

Amiloride

George CF. Amiloride handling in renal failure. Br J Clin Pharmacol. 1980;9:94-5.

Spahn H, Reuter K, Mutschler E, et al. Pharmacokinetics of amiloride in renal and hepatic disease. Eur J Clin Pharmacol. 1987;33:493-8.

Bumetanide

Lau HS, Hyneck ML, Berardi RR, et al. Kinetics, dynamics, and bioavailability of bumetanide in healthy subjects and patients with chronic renal failure. Clin Pharmacol Ther. 1986;39:635-45.

Pentikainen PJ, Pasternack A, Lampainen E, et al. Bumetanide kinetics in renal failure. Clin Pharmacol Ther. 1985;37:582-8.

Ward A, Heel RC. Bumetanide: a review of its pharmacodynamic and pharmacokinetic properties and therapeutic use. Drugs. 1984;28:426-64.

Chlorthalidone

Mulley BA, Parr GD, Rye RM. Pharmacokinetics of chlorthalidone. Eur J Clin Pharmacol. 1980;17:203-7.

Ethacrynic Acid

Pillary VK, Schwartz FD, Aimi K, et al. Transient and permanent deafness following treatment of ethacrynic acid in renal failure. Lancet. 1969;1:77-9.

Furosemide

Boles LL, Shoenwald RD. Furosemide (frusemide): a pharmacokinetic/pharmacodynamic review (Part 1). Clin Pharmacokinet. 1990;18:381-408.

Traeger A, Stein G, Sperschneider H, et al. Pharmacokinetic and pharmacodynamic effects of furosemide in patients with impaired renal function. Int J Clin Pharmacol Ther Toxicol. 1984;22:481-6.

Indapamide

Chaffman M, Heel RC, Brogden RN, et al. Indapamide: a review of its pharmacodynamic properties and therapeutic efficacy in hypertension. Drugs. 1984;28:189-235.

Metolazone

No references

Piretanide

Clissold SP, Brogden RN. Piretinide: a preliminary review of its pharmacodynamic and pharmacokinetic properties, and therapeutic efficacy. Drugs. 1985;29:489-530.

Marsh, JD, Smith TW. Piretanide: a loop-active diuretic; pharmacology, therapeutic efficacy and adverse effects. Pharmacotherapy. 1984;4:170-80.

Walter U, Rockel A, Lahn W, et al. Pharmacokinetics of the loop diuretic piretinide in renal failure. Eur J Clin Pharmacol. 1985;29:337-43.

Spironolactone

Morris RG, Frewin DB, Taylor WB, et al. The effect of renal and hepatic impairment of spironolactone on digoxin immunoassays. Eur J Clin Pharmacol. 1988;34:233-9.

Skluth HA, Gums JG. Spironolactone: a re-examination. Drug Intell Clin Pharm. 1990;24:52-9.

Thiazides

Niemeyer C, Hasenfub G, Wais U, et al. Pharmacokinetics of hydrochlorothiazide in relation to renal function. Eur J Clin Pharmacol. 1983;24:61-5.

Torasemide

Dunn DJ, Fitton A, Brogden RN. Torasemide: an update of its pharmacological properties and therapeutic efficacy. Drugs. 1995;49:121-42.

Friedel HA, Buckley MM. Torasemide: a review of its pharmacological properties and therapeutic potential drugs. Drugs. 1991;41:81-103.

Gehr TWB, Rudy DW, Matzke GR, et al. The pharmacokinetics of intravenous and oral torasemide in patients with chronic renal insufficiency. Clin Pharmacol Ther. 1994;56:31-8.

Kramer BK, Schwab A, Braun N, et al. Pharmacokinetics of torasemide and its metabolites in end-stage renal disease. Eur J Clin Pharmacol. 1994;47:157-9.

Triamterene

[Anonymous]. Triamterene and the kidney [Editorial]. Lancet. 1986;1:424.

Fairley KF, Woo KT, Birch DF, et al. Triamterene-induced crystalluria and cylinduria: clinical and experimental studies. Clin Nephrol. 1986;26:169-73.

MISCELLANEOUS CARDIAC DRUGS

Amrinone

Bottorff MB, Rutledge DR, Pieper JA. Evaluation of intravenous amrinone: the first of a new class of positive inotropic agents with vasodilator properties. Pharmacotherapy. 1984;5:227-36.

Dobutamine

Lawless CE, Loeb HS. Pharmacokinetics and pharmacodynamics of Dobutamine. In: Chatterjee ED, ed. Dobutamine. New York: NCM Publishers; 1989:33-47.

Majerus TC, Dasta JF, Bauman JL, et al. Dobutamine: ten years later. Pharmacotherapy. 1989;9:245-59.

Midodrine

McTavish D, Goa KL. Midodrine: a review of its pharmacological properties and therapeutic use in orthostatic hypotension and secondary hypotensive disorders. Drugs. 1989;38:757-77.

Milrinone

Larsson R, Liedholm H, Andersson KE, et al. Pharmacokinetics and effects on blood pressure of a single oral dose of milrinone in healthy subjects and in patients with renal impairment. Eur J Clin Pharmacol. 1986;29:549-53.

Young RA, Ward A. Milrinone: a preliminary review of its pharmacological properties and therapeutic use. Drugs. 1988;36:158-92.

NITRATES

Isosorbide

Evers J, Bonn R, Boertz A, et al. Pharmacokinetics of isosorbide dinitrate, isosorbide-2-nitrate and isosorbide-5-nitrate in renal insufficiency after repeated oral dosage. Klin Wochenschr. 1989;67:342-8.

Fung HL. Pharmacokinetics and pharmacodynamics of organic nitrates. Am J Cardiol. 1987;60:4H-9H.

Todd PA, Goa KL, Langtry HD. Transdermal nitroglycerin (glyceryl tri-nitrate): a review of its pharmacology and therapeutic use. Drugs. 1990;40:880-902.

Nitroglycerin

Fung HL. Pharmacokinetics and pharmacodynamics of organic nitrates. Am J Cardiol. 1987;60:4H-9H.
Todd PA, Goa KL, Langtry HD. Transdermal nitroglycerin (glyceryl tri-nitrate): a review of its pharmacology and therapeutic use. Drugs. 1990;40:880-902.

Antimicrobial Agents

ANTIBACTERIAL ANTIBIOTICS

AMINOGLYCOSIDE ANTIBIOTICS

Amikacin

French MA, Cerra FB, Plaut ME, et al. Amikacin and gentamicin accumulation pharmacokinetics and nephrotoxicity in critically ill patients. Antimicrob Agents Chemother. 1981;19:147-52.
Regeur L, Colding H, Jensen H, et al. Pharmacokinetics of amikacin during hemodialysis and peritoneal dialysis. Antimicrob Agents Chemother. 1977;11:214-8.

Gentamicin

De Paepe M, Lameire N, Belpaire F, et al. Peritoneal pharmacokinetics of gentamicin in man. Clin Nephrol. 1983;19:107-9.
Pancorbo S, Comty C. Pharmacokinetics of gentamicin in patients undergoing continuous ambulatory peritoneal dialysis. Antimicrob Agents Chemother. 1981;19:605-7.
Thompson MI, Russo ME, Saxon BJ, et al. Gentamicin inactivation by piperacillin or carbenicillin in patients with end-stage renal disease. Antimicrob Agents Chemother. 1983;21:268-73.

Kanamycin

No references

Netilmicin

Luft FC, Brannon DR, Stropes LL, et al. Pharmacokinetics of netilmicin in patients with renal impairment in patients on dialysis. Antimicrob Agents Chemother. 1983;14:403-7.

Streptomycin

No references

Tobramycin

Aarons L, Vozeh S, Wenk M, et al. Population pharmacokinetics of tobramycin. Br J Clin Pharmacokinet. 1989;28:305-14.

Brogden RN, Pender RM, Sawyer TM, et al. Tobramycin: a review of its antibacterial and pharmacokinetic properties and therapeutic use. Drugs. 1976;12:166-200.

Bunke CM, Aronoff GR, Brier ME, et al. Tobramycin kinetics during continuous ambulatory peritoneal dialysis. Clin Pharmacol Ther. 1983;34:110-6.

CEPHALOSPORIN ANTIBIOTICS

Cefaclor

Spyker DA, Gober LL, Scheld WM, et al. Pharmacokinetics of cefaclor in renal failure: effects of multiple doses and hemodialysis. Antimicrob Agents Chemother. 1982;21:278-81.

Cefadroxil

Cutler RE, Blair AD, Kelly MR. Cefadroxil kinetics in patients with renal insufficiency. Clin Pharmacol Ther. 1979;25(Suppl):514-21.

Leroy A, Humbert G, Godin M, et al. Pharmacokinetics of cefoxadril in patients with impaired renal function. Antimicrob Chemother. 1982;10(Suppl B):39-46.

Cefamandole

Czerwinski A, Fenderson J. Pharmacokinetics of cefamandole in patients with renal impairment. Antimicrob Agents Chemother. 1979;15:161-4.

Gambertoglio JG, Aziz NS, Lin ET, et al. Cefamandole kinetics in uremic patients undergoing hemodialysis. Clin Pharmacol Ther. 1979;26:592-9.

Pancorbo S, Comty C. Pharmacokinetics of cefamandole in patients undergoing continuous ambulatory peritoneal dialysis. Perit Dial Bull. 1983;2:135-7.

Cefazolin

Brogard JM, Pinget M, Brandt C, et al. Pharmacokinetics of cefazolin in patients with renal failure: special reference to hemodialysis. J Clin Pharmacol. 1977;17:225-30.

Hiner LB, Baluarte HJ, Polinsky MS, et al. Cefazolin in children with renal insufficiency. J Pediatr. 1980;96:335-9.

Kaye D, Wenger N, Agarwal B. Pharmacology of intraperitoneal cefazolin in patients undergoing peritoneal dialysis. Antimicrob Agents Chemother. 1978;14:318-21.

Cefepime

Barbhaiya RH, Forgue ST, Gleason CR, et al. Pharmacokinetics of cefepime after single and multiple intravenous administration in healthy subjects. Antimicrob Agents Chemother. 1992;36:552-7.

Barbhaiya RH, Knupp CA, Forgue ST, et al. Pharmacokinetics of cefepime in subjects with renal insufficiency. Clin Pharm Ther. 1990;48:268-76.

Barbhaiya RH, Knupp CA, Pfeffer M, et al. Pharmacokinetics of cefepime in patients undergoing continuous ambulatory peritoneal dialysis. Antimicrob Agents Chemother. 1992;36:1387-91.

Cefixime

Faulkner RD, Bohaychuk W, Lance RA, et al. Pharmacokinetics of cefixime in the young and elderly. J Antimicrob Chemother. 1988;21:787-94.

Guay DR, Meatherall RC, Harding GK, et al. Pharmacokinetics of cefixime (CL284,635FK027) in healthy subjects and patients with renal insufficiency. Antimicrob Agents Chemother. 1986;30:485-90.

Cefmenoxime

Konish, K. Pharmacokinetics of cefmenoxime in patients with impaired renal function and in those undergoing hemodialysis. Antimicrob Agents Chemother. 1986;30:901-5.

Cefmetazole

Halstenson CE, Guay DR, Opsahl JA, et al. Disposition of cefmetazole in healthy volunteers and patients with impaired renal function. Antimicrob Agents Chemother. 1990;34:519-23.

Cefonicid

Barriere SL, Gambertoglio, JG, Alexander DP, et al. Pharmacokinetic disposition of cefonicid in patients with renal failure and receiving hemodialysis. Rev Infect Dis. 1984;6(Suppl 4):S809-15.

Blair AD, Maxwell BM, Forland SC, et al. Cefonicid kinetics in subjects with normal and impaired renal function. Clin Pharmacol Ther. 1984;35:798-803.

Cefoperazone

Greenfield RA, Gerber AU, Craig WA. Pharmacokinetics of cefoperazone in patients with normal and impaired hepatic and renal function. Rev Infect Dis. 1983;5:S127-36.

Keller E, Jansen A, Pelz K, et al. Intraperitoneal and intravenous cefoperazone kinetics during continuous ambulatory peritoneal dialysis. Clin Pharmocol Ther. 1984;35:208-13.

Spyker DA, Richmond JD, Scheld WM, et al. Pharmacokinetics of multiple-dose cefoperazone in hemodialysis patients. Am J Nephrol. 1985;5:355-60.

Trollfors B, Ahlemen J, Alestig K. Renal function during cefoperazone treatment. J Antimicrob Chemother. 1982;9:485-7.

Ceforanide

Estey EH, Weaver SS, LeBlanc BM, et al. Ceforanide kinetics. Clin Pharmacol Ther. 1981;30:398-403.

Hawkins SS, Alford RH, Stone WJ, et al. Ceforanide kinetics in renal insufficiency. Clin Pharmacol Ther. 1981;30:468-74.

Cefotaxime

Albin HC, Demotes-Mainard FM, Bouchett JL, et al. Pharmacokinetics of intravenous and intraperitoneal cefotaxime in chronic ambulatory peritoneal dialysis. Clin Pharmacol Ther. 1985;38:285-9.

Doluisio JT. Clinical pharmacokinetics of cefotaxime in patients with normal and reduced renal function. Rev Infect Dis. 1982;4(Suppl):S33-45.

Ings RM, Fillastre JP, Godin M, et al. The pharmacokinetics of cefotaxime and its metabolites in subjects with normal and impaired renal function. Rev Infect Dis. 1982;4(Suppl):S379-91.

Peterson J, Stewart RD, Catto GR, et al. Pharmacokinetics of intraperitoneal cefotaxime treatment of peritonitis in patients on continuous ambulatory peritoneal dialysis. Nephron. 1985;40:79-82.

Rodondi LC, Flaherty JF, Schoenfeld P, et al. Influence of coadministration on the pharmacokinetics of mezlocillin and cefotaxime in healthy volunteers and in patients with renal failure. Clin Pharmacol Ther. 1989;45:527-34.

Cefotetan

Browning MJ, Hoh HA, White LD, et al. Pharmacokinetics of cefoteten in patients with end-stage renal failure on maintenence dialysis. J Antimicrob Chemother. 1986;18:103-6.

Ohkawa M, Hirano S, Tokunaga S, et al. Pharmacokinetics of cefotetan in normal subjects and patients with impaired renal function. Antimicrob Agents Chemother. 1983;23:31-5.

Ward A, Richards DM. Cefoteten: a review of its antimicrobial activity, pharmacokinetic properties and therapeutic uses. Drugs. 1985;30:382-426.

Cefoxitin

Arvidsson A, Alvan G, Tranaeue A, et al. Pharmacokinetic studies of cefoxitin in continuous ambulatory peritoneal dialysis. Eur J Clin Pharmacol. 1985;28:333-7.

Brogden RN, Heel RC, Speight TM, et al. Cefoxitin: a review of its antibacterial activity, pharmacological properties and therapeutic use. Drugs. 1979;17:1-37.

Fillastre JP, Leroy A, Godin M, et al. Pharmacokinetics of cefoxitin sodium in normal subjects and in uraemic patients. J Antimicrob Chemother. 1978;4(Suppl B):79-83.

Cefpodoxime

Borin MT, Hughes GS, Kelloway JS, et al. Disposition of cefpodoxime proxetil in hemodialysis patients. J Clin Pharmacol. 1992;32:1038-44.

St. Peter JV, Borin MT, Hughes GS, et al. Disposition of cefpodoxime proxetil in healthy volunteers and patients with impaired renal function. Antimicrob Agents Chemother. 1992;36:126-31.

Cefprozil

Shyu WC, Pittmen KA, Wilber RB, et al. Pharmacokinetics of cefprozil in healthy subjects and patients with renal impairment. J Clin Pharmacol. 1991;31:362-71.

Ceftazidime

Ackerman BH, Ross J, Tofte RW, et al. Effect of decreased renal function on the pharmacokinetics of ceftazidime. Antimicrob Agents Chemother. 1984;25:785-6.

Lin MS, Wang LS, Huang JD. Single and multiple dose pharmacokinetics of ceftazidime in infected patients with varying degrees of renal function. J Clin Pharmacol. 1989;29:331-7.

Tourkantonis A, Nikolaidis P. Pharmacokinetics of ceftazidime in patients undergoing peritoneal dialysis. J Antimicrob Chemother. 1983;12(Suppl A):263-7.

Ceftibuten

Barr WH, Lin CC, Radwanski E, et al. The pharmacokinetics of ceftibuten in humans. Diag Microbiol Infect Dis. 1991;14:93-100.

Kelloway JS, Awni WM, Lin CC, et al. Pharmacokinetics of ceftibutin-*cis* and its trans-metabolite in healthy volunteers and in patients with chronic renal insufficiency. Antimicrob Agents Chemother. 1991;35:2267-74.

Ceftizoxime

Gross ML, Somani P, Ribner BS, et al. Ceftizoxime elimination kinetics in continuous ambulatory peritoneal dialysis. Clin Pharmacol Ther. 1983;34:673-80.

Kowalsky SF, Echols RM, Venezia AR, et al. Pharmacokinetics of ceftizoxime in subjects with various degrees of renal function. Antimicrob Agents Chemother. 1983;24:151-5.

Ceftriaxone

Stoeckel K, Koup JR. Pharmacokinetics of ceftriaxone in patients with renal and liver insufficiency and correlations with a physiologic nonlinear protein binding model. Am J Med. 1984;77:26-32.

Ti TY, Fortin L, Kreeft JH, et al. Kinetics disposition of intravenous ceftriaxone in normal subjects and patients with renal failure on hemodialysis or peritoneal dialysis. Antimicrob Agents Chemother. 1984;25:83-7.

Cefuroxime Axetil

Chan MK, Browning AK, Poole CJ, et al. Cefuroxime pharmacokinetics in continuous and intermittent peritoneal dialysis. Nephron. 1985;41:161-5.

Walstad RA, Nilsen OG, Berg KJ. Pharmacokinetics and clinical effects of cefuroxime in patients with severe renal insufficiency. Eur J Clin Pharmacol. 1983;24:391-8.

Cefuroxime Sodium

No references

Cephalexin

Bailey RR, Gower PE, Dash CH. The effects of impairment of renal function and hemodialysis on serum and urine levels of cephalexin. Postgrad Med J. 1970;46(Suppl):60-4.

Bunke CM, Aronoff GR, Brier ME, et al. Cefazolin and cephalexin kinetics in continuous ambulatory peritoneal dialysis. Clin Pharmacol Ther. 1983;33:66-72.

Drew PJ, Casewell MW, Desai N, et al. Cephalexin for the oral treatment of CAPD peritonitis. J Antimicrob Chemother. 1984;13:153-9.

Cephalothin

Munch R, Steurer J, Luthy R, et al. Serum and dialyzate concentrations of intraperitoneal cephalothin in patients undergoing continuous ambulatory peritoneal dialysis. Clin Nephrol. 1983;20:40-3.

Rankin LI, Swain RR, Luft FC. Effect of cephalothin on measurement of creatinine concentration. Antimicrob Agents Chemother. 1979;15:666-9.

Venuto RC, Plaut M. Cephalothin handling in patients undergoing hemodialysis. Antimicrob Agents Chemother. 1970;10:50-2.

Cephapirin

Bergan T, Orjavik O, Brodwall EK. Pharmacokinetics of cephapirin in patients with normal and impaired renal function. Arzneimittelforschung. 1981;31:1773-6.

McCloskey RV, Terry EE, McCracken AW, et al. Effect of hemodialysis and renal failure on serum and urine concentrations of cephapirin sodium. Antimicrob Agents Chemother. 1972;1:90-3.

Cephradine

Johnson CA, Welling PG, Zimmerman SW. Pharmacokinetics of oral cephradine in continuous ambulatory peritoneal dialysis patients. Nephron. 1984;38:57-61.

Searle M, Raman GV. Oral treatment of peritonitis complicating continuous ambulatory peritoneal dialysis. Clin Nephrol. 1985;23:241-4.

Solomon AE, Briggs JD. The administration of cefradine to patients in renal failure. Br J Clin Pharmacol. 1975;2:443-8.

Moxalactam

Aronoff GR, Sloan RS, Mong SA, et al. Moxalactam pharmacokinetics during hemodialysis. Antimicrob Agents Chemother. 1981;19:575-7.

Aronoff GR, Sloan RS, Luft FC. Pharmacokinetics of moxalactam in patients with normal and impaired renal function. J Infect Dis. 1985;23:241-4.

Jones TE, Milne RW, Mudaliar Y, et al. Moxalactam kinetics during continuous ambulatory peritoneal dialysis after intraperitoneal administration. Antimicrob Agents Chemother. 1985;28:293-8.

MISCELLANEOUS ANTIBACTERIAL ANTIBIOTICS

Azithromycin

Golper TA, Gleason JR, Vincent HH, et al. Drug removal during high efficiency and high flux hemodialysis. Contemp Iss Nephrol. 1993;27:175-208.

Hoffler D, Koeppe P, Paeske B. Pharmacokinetics of azithromycin in normal and impaired renal function. Infection. 1995;23:356-61.

Keane WF, Everett ED, Golper TA, et al. Peritoneal dialysis-related peritonitis treatment recommendations: 1993 update. Perit Dial Int. 1993;13:14-28.

Lalak NJ, Morris DL. Azithromycin clinical pharmacokinetics. Clin Pharmacokinet. 1993;25:370-4.

St. Peter WL, Redic-Kill KA, Haltenson CE. Clinical pharmacokinetics of antibiotics in patients with impaired renal function. Clin Pharmacokinet. 1992;22:169-210.

Aztreonam

Brogden RN, Heel RC. Aztreonam: a review of its antibacterial activity, pharmacokinetic properties and therapeutic use. Drugs. 1986;31:96-130.

Fillastre JP, Leroy A, Baudoin C, et al. Pharmacokinetics of aztreonam in patients with chronic renal failure. Clin Pharmacokinet. 1985;10:91-100.

Gerig JS, Bolton ND, Swabb EA, et al. Effect of hemodialysis and peritoneal dialysis on aztreonam pharmacokinetics. Kidney Int. 1984;26:308-18.

Golper TA, Gleason JR, Vincent HH, et al. Drug removal during high efficiency and high flux hemodialysis. Contemp Iss Nephrol. 1993;27:175-208.

Keane WF, Everett ED, Golper TA, et al. Peritoneal dialysis-related peritonitis treatment recommendations: 1993 update. Perit Dial Int. 1993;13:14-28.

St. Peter WL, Redic-Kill KA, Haltenson CE. Clinical pharmacokinetics of antibiotics in patients with impaired renal function. Clin Pharmacokinet. 1992;22:169-210.

Chloramphenicol

Ambrose PJ. Clinical pharmacokinetics of chloraphenicol and chloramphenicol succinate. Clin Pharmacokinet. 1984;9:222-38.

Golper TA, Gleason JR, Vincent HH, et al. Drug removal during high efficiency and high flux hemodialysis. Contemp Iss Nephrol. 1993;27:175-208.

Grafnetterova J, Vodrazka Z, Jandova D, et al. The binding of chloramphenicol to serum proteins in patients with chronic renal insufficiency. Clin Nephrol. 1976;6:448-50.

Keane WF, Everett ED, Golper TA, et al. Peritoneal dialysis-related peritonitis treatment recommendations: 1993 update. Perit Dial Int. 1993;13:14-28.

Slaughter RL, Cerra FB, Koup JR. Effect of hemodialysis on total body clearance of chloramphenicol. Am J Hosp Pharm. 1980;37:1083-6.

St. Peter WL, Redic-Kill KA, Haltenson CE. Clinical pharmacokinetics of antibiotics in patients with impaired renal function. Clin Pharmacokinet. 1992;22:169-210.

Cilastin

Golper TA, Gleason JR, Vincent HH, et al. Drug removal during high efficiency and high flux hemodialysis. Contemp Iss Nephrol. 1993;27:175-208.

Keane WF, Everett ED, Golper TA, et al. Peritoneal dialysis-related peritonitis treatment recommendations: 1993 update. Perit Dial Int. 1993;13:14-28.

St. Peter WL, Redic-Kill KA, Haltenson CE. Clinical pharmacokinetics of antibiotics in patients with impaired renal function. Clin Pharmacokinet. 1992;22:169-210.

Clarithromycin

Chu SY, Sennello LT, Bunnell ST, et al. Pharmacokinetics of clarithromycin, a new macrolide after single ascending oral doses. Antimicrob Agents Chemother. 1992;36:2447-53.

Ferrero JL, Bopp BA, Marsh KC, et al. Metabolism and disposition of clarithromycin in man. Drug Metab Dispos Biol Fate Chem. 1990;18:441-6.

Golper TA, Gleason JR, Vincent HH, et al. Drug removal during high efficiency and high flux hemodialysis. Contemp Iss Nephrol. 1993;27:175-208.

Keane WF, Everett ED, Golper TA, et al. Peritoneal dialysis-related peritonitis treatment recommendations: 1993 update. Perit Dial Int. 1993;13:14-28.

St. Peter WL, Redic-Kill KA, Haltenson CE. Clinical pharmacokinetics of antibiotics in patients with impaired renal function. Clin Pharmacokinet. 1992;22:169-210.

Clavulanic Acid

Adam D, de Visser I, Koeppe P. Pharmacokinetics of amoxicillin and clavulanic acid administered alone and in combination. Antimicrob Agents Chemother. 1982;22:353-7.

Dalet F, Amado E, Cabrera E, et al. Pharmacokinetics of the combination of ticarcillin with clavulanic acid in renal insufficiency. J Antimicrob Chemother. 1986;17(Suppl C):57-64.

Davies BE, Boon R, Horton R, et al. Pharmacokinetics of amoxicillin and clavulanic acid in hemodialysis patients following intravenous administration of Augmentin. Br J Clin Pharmacol. 1988;26:385-90.

Golper TA, Gleason JR, Vincent HH, et al. Drug removal during high efficiency and high flux hemodialysis. Contemp Iss Nephrol. 1993;27:175-208.

Horber FF, Frey FJ, Descoeudres C, Murray AT, Reubi FC. Differential effect of impaired renal function on the kinetics of clavulanic acid and amoxicillin. Antimicrob Agents Chemother. 1986;29:614-619.

Jackson D, Cooper DL, Filer CW, et al. Augmentin absorption, excretion and pharmacokientic studies in man. Postgrad Med. 1984;76(Suppl):51-70.

Keane WF, Everett ED, Golper TA, et al. Peritoneal dialysis-related peritonitis treatment recommendations: 1993 update. Perit Dial Int. 1993;13:14-28.

Slaughter RL, Kohli R, Brass C. Effects of hemodialysis on the pharmacokinetics of amoxicillin/clavulanic acid and combination. Ther Drug Monit. 1984;6:424-7.

St. Peter WL, Redic-Kill KA, Haltenson CE. Clinical pharmacokinetics of antibiotics in patients with impaired renal function. Clin Pharmacokinet. 1992;22:169-210.

Clindamycin

Golper TA, Gleason JR, Vincent HH, et al. Drug removal during high efficiency and high flux hemodialysis. Contemp Iss Nephrol. 1993;27:175-208.

Golper TA, Sewell DL, Fisher PB, et al. Incomplete activation of intraperitoneal clindamycin phosphate during peritoneal dialysis. Am J Nephrol. 1984;6:38-42.

Keane WF, Everett ED, Golper TA, et al. Peritoneal dialysis-related peritonitis treatment recommendations: 1993 update. Perit Dial Int. 1993;13:14-28.

Roberts A, Eastwood J, Gower P, et al. Serum and plasma concentrations of clindamycin following a single intramuscular injection of clindamycin phosphate in maintenance hemodialysis patients and normal subjects. Eur J Pharmacol. 1978;14:435-9.

St. Peter WL, Redic-Kill KA, Haltenson CE. Clinical pharmacokinetics of antibiotics in patients with impaired renal function. Clin Pharmacokinet. 1992;22:169-210.

Clofazamine

Holdiness MR. Clinical pharmacokinetics of clofazamine. Clin Pharmacokinet. 1989;16:74-85.

Dapsone

Edstein MD, Rieckmann KH, Veenendaal JR. Multiple-dose pharmacokinetics and in vitro antimalarial activity of dapsone plus pyrimethamine (Maloprim) in man. Br J Clin Pharmacol. 1990;30:259-65.

Zuidema J, Hilbers-Modderman ESM, Merkus FWHM. Clinical pharmacokinetics of dapsone. Clin Pharmacokinet. 1986;11:299-315.

Dirithromycin

Ripley ED, Sica DA, Gehr TW, et al. Dirithryomycin pharmacokinetics in hemodialysis and chronic renal failure [Abstract]. Clin Pharmacol Ther. 1992;51:137.

Sides GD, Cerimele BJ, Black HR, et al. Pharmacokinetics of dirithromycin. J Antimicrob Chemother. 1993;31(Suppl C):65-75.

Erythromycin

Golper TA, Gleason JR, Vincent HH, et al. Drug removal during high efficiency and high flux hemodialysis. Contemp Iss Nephrol. 1993;27:175-208.

Kanfer A, Stamatakis G, Torlotin JC, et al. Changes in erythromycin pharmacokinetics induced by renal failure. Clin Nephrol. 1987;27:147-50.

Keane WF, Everett ED, Golper TA, et al. Peritoneal dialysis-related peritonitis treatment recommendations: 1993 update. Perit Dial Int. 1993;13:14-28.

Krobath PD, McNeil MA, Kreeger A, et al. Hearing loss and erythromycin pharmacokinetics in a patient receiving hemodialysis. Arch Intern Med. 1983;143:1263-5.

Welling PG, Craig WA. Pharmacokinetics of intravenous erythromycin. J Pharm Sci. 1978;17:1057-9.

St. Peter WL, Redic-Kill KA, Haltenson CE. Clinical pharmacokinetics of antibiotics in patients with impaired renal function. Clin Pharmacokinet. 1992;22:169-210.

Imipenem

Gibson TP, Demetriades JL, Bland JA. Imipenem/cilastin: pharmacokinetic profile in renal insufficiency. Am J Med. 1985;78:(Suppl 6A):54-61.

Golper TA, Gleason JR, Vincent HH, et al. Drug removal during high efficiency and high flux hemodialysis. Contemp Iss Nephrol. 1993;27:175-208.

Keane WF, Everett ED, Golper TA, et al. Peritoneal dialysis-related peritonitis treatment recommendations: 1993 update. Perit Dial Int. 1993;13:14-28.

Konishi K, Suzuki H, Saruta T, et al. Removal of imipenem and cilastin by hemodialysis in patients with end-stage renal failure. Antimicrob Agents Chemother. 1991;35:1616-20.

Mueller BA, Scarim SK, Macias WL. Comparison of imipenem pharmacokinetics in patients with acute or chronic renal failure treated with continuous hemofiltration. Am J Kid Dis. 1993;21:172-9.

St. Peter WL, Redic-Kill KA, Haltenson CE. Clinical pharmacokinetics of antibiotics in patients with impaired renal function. Clin Pharmacokinet. 1992;22:169-210.

Verbist L, Verpooten GA, Giuliano RA, et al. Pharmacokinetics and tolerance after repeated doses of imipenem/cilastin in patients with severe renal failure. J Antimicrob Chemother. 1986;18(Suppl E):115-20.

Lincomycin

Golper TA, Gleason JR, Vincent HH, et al. Drug removal during high efficiency and high flux hemodialysis. Contemp Iss Nephrol. 1993;27:175-208.

Keane WF, Everett ED, Golper TA, et al. Peritoneal dialysis-related peritonitis treatment recommendations: 1993 update. Perit Dial Int. 1993;13:14-28.

Malacoff RF, Finkelstein FO, Andriole VT. Effect of peritoneal dialysis on serum levels of tobramycin and lincomycin. Antimicrob Agents Chemother. 1975;8:574-80.

St. Peter WL, Redic-Kill KA, Haltenson CE. Clinical pharmacokinetics of antibiotics in patients with impaired renal function. Clin Pharmacokinet. 1992;22:169-210.

Loracarbef

Therasse DG, Farlow DS, Davidson RL, et al. Effects of renal dysfunction on the pharmacokinetics of loracarbef. Clin Pharmacol Ther. 1993;54:311-6.

Meropenem

Chimata M, Vagase M, Suzuki Y, et al. Pharmacokinetics of meropenem in patients with various degrees of renal function including patients with end-stage renal disease. Antimicrob Agents Chemother. 1993;37:229-33.

Christensson BA, Nilsson-Ehle I, Hutchinson M, et al. Pharmacokinetics of meropenem in subjects with various degrees of renal impairment. Antimicrob Agents Chemother. 1992;36:1532-37.

Golper TA, Gleason JR, Vincent HH, et al. Drug removal during high efficiency and high flux hemodialysis. Contemp Iss Nephrol. 1993;27:175-208.

Keane WF, Everett ED, Golper TA, et al. Peritoneal dialysis-related peritonitis treatment recommendations: 1993 update. Perit Dial Int. 1993;13:14-28.

St. Peter WL, Redic-Kill KA, Haltenson CE. Clinical pharmacokinetics of antibiotics in patients with impaired renal function. Clin Pharmacokinet. 1992;22:169-210.

Methenamine Mandelate

Golper TA, Gleason JR, Vincent HH, et al. Drug removal during high efficiency and high flux hemodialysis. Contemp Iss Nephrol. 1993;27:175-208.

Hamilton-Miller JM, Brumfitt W. Methenamine and its salts as urinary tract antiseptics: variables affecting the antibacterial activity of formaldehyde, mandelic acid, and hippuric acid in vitro. Invest Urol. 1977;14:287-91.

Keane WF, Everett ED, Golper TA, et al. Peritoneal dialysis-related peritonitis treatment recommendations: 1993 update. Perit Dial Int. 1993;13:14-28.

St. Peter WL, Redic-Kill KA, Haltenson CE. Clinical pharmacokinetics of antibiotics in patients with impaired renal function. Clin Pharmacokinet. 1992;22:169-210.

Metronidazole

Golper TA, Gleason JR, Vincent HH, et al. Drug removal during high efficiency and high flux hemodialysis. Contemp Iss Nephrol. 1993;27:175-208.

Guay DR, Meatherall RC, Baxter H, et al. Pharmacokinetics of metronidazole in patients undergoing continuous ambulatory peritoneal dialysis. Antimicrob Agents Chemother. 1984;25:306-10.

Houghton GW, Dennis MJ, Gabriel P. Pharmacokinetics of metronidazole in patients with varying degrees of renal failure. Br J Clin Pharmacol. 1985;19:203-9.

Keane WF, Everett ED, Golper TA, et al. Peritoneal dialysis-related peritonitis treatment recommendations: 1993 update. Perit Dial Int. 1993;13:14-28.

Lau AH, Chang CW, Sabatini S. Hemodialysis clearance of metronidazole and its metabolites. Antimicrob Agents Chemother. 1986;29:235-8.

St. Peter WL, Redic-Kill KA, Haltenson CE. Clinical pharmacokinetics of antibiotics in patients with impaired renal function. Clin Pharmacokinet. 1992;22:169-210.

Nitrofurantoin

Conklin JD. The pharmacokinetics of nitrofurantoin and its related bioavailability. Antibiot Chemother. 1978;25:233-52.

Golper TA, Gleason JR, Vincent HH, et al. Drug removal during high efficiency and high flux hemodialysis. Contemp Iss Nephrol. 1993;27:175-208.

Keane WF, Everett ED, Golper TA, et al. Peritoneal dialysis-related peritonitis treatment recommendations: 1993 update. Perit Dial Int. 1993;13:14-28.

Liedtke RK, Ebel S, Missler B, et al. Single-dose pharmacokinetics of macrocrystalline nitrofurantoin formulations. Arzneimittel-forschung. 1980;20:833-6.

St. Peter WL, Redic-Kill KA, Haltenson CE. Clinical pharmacokinetics of antibiotics in patients with impaired renal function. Clin Pharmacokinet. 1992;22:169-210.

Toole JF, Parrish ML. Nitrofurantoin polyneuropathy. Neurology. 1973;23:554-9.

Spectinomycin

Golper TA, Gleason JR, Vincent HH, et al. Drug removal during high efficiency and high flux hemodialysis. Contemp Iss Nephrol. 1993;27:175-208.

Keane WF, Everett ED, Golper TA, et al. Peritoneal dialysis-related peritonitis treatment recommendations: 1993 update. Perit Dial Int. 1993;13:14-28.

Kusumi R, Metzler C, Fass R. Pharmacokinetics of spectinomycin in volunteers with renal insufficiency. Chemotherapy. 1981;27:95-8.

St. Peter WL, Redic-Kill KA, Haltenson CE. Clinical pharmacokinetics of antibiotics in patients with impaired renal function. Clin Pharmacokinet. 1992;22:169-210.

Sulbactam

Golper TA, Gleason JR, Vincent HH, et al. Drug removal during high efficiency and high flux hemodialysis. Contemp Iss Nephrol. 1993;27:175-208.

Keane WF, Everett ED, Golper TA, et al. Peritoneal dialysis-related peritonitis treatment recommendations: 1993 update. Perit Dial Int. 1993;13:14-28.

Reitberg DP, Marble DA, Schultz RW, et al. Pharmacokinetics of cefoperazone (2g) and sulbactam (1g) coadministered to subjects with normal renal function, patients with decreased renal function, and patients with end-stage renal disease on dialysis. Antimicrob Agents Chemother. 1988;32:503-9.

St. Peter WL, Redic-Kill KA, Haltenson CE. Clinical pharmacokinetics of antibiotics in patients with impaired renal function. Clin Pharmacokinet. 1992;22:169-210.

Wright N, Wise R. Elimination of sulbactam alone and combined with ampicillin in patients with renal dysfunction. J Antimicrob Chemother. 1983;11:583-7.

Sulfamethoxazole

Berglund F, Killander J, Pompeius R. Effect of trimethoprim-sulfamethoxazole on renal excretion of creatinine in man. J Urol. 1975;114:802-8.

Golper TA, Gleason JR, Vincent HH, et al. Drug removal during high efficiency and high flux hemodialysis. Contemp Iss Nephrol. 1993;27:175-208.

Halstenson CE, Blevins RB, Salem NG, et al. Trimethoprim-sulfamethoxazole pharmacokinetics during continuous ambulatory peritoneal dialysis. Clin Nephrol. 1984;22:239-43.

Keane WF, Everett ED, Golper TA, et al. Peritoneal dialysis-related peritonitis treatment recommendations: 1993 update. Perit Dial Int. 1993;13:14-28.

Siber GR, Gorham CC, Ericson JF, et al. Pharmacokinetics of intravenous trimethoprim-sulfamethoxazole in children and adults with normal and impaired renal function. Rev Infect Dis. 1982;4:566-78.

St. Peter WL, Redic-Kill KA, Haltenson CE. Clinical pharmacokinetics of antibiotics in patients with impaired renal function. Clin Pharmacokinet. 1992;22:169-210.

Sulfisoxazole

No references

Tazobactam

Golper TA, Gleason JR, Vincent HH, et al. Drug removal during high efficiency and high flux hemodialysis. Contemp Iss Nephrol. 1993;27:175-208.

Halstenson CE, Wong MO, Johnson CA, et al. Pharmacokinetics of tazobactam M1 metabolite after administration of piperacillin/tazobactam in subjects with renal impairment. J Clin Pharmacol. 1994;34:1208-17.

Johnson CA, Haltenson CE, Kelloway BE, et al. Single dose pharmacokinetics of piperacillin and tazobactam in patients with renal disease. Clin Pharmacol Ther. 1992;51:32-41.

Keane WF, Everett ED, Golper TA, et al. Peritoneal dialysis-related peritonitis treatment recommendations: 1993 update. Perit Dial Int. 1993;13:14-28.

Sorgel F, Kinzig M. The chemistry, pharmacokinetics and tissue distribution of piperacillin/tazobactam. J Antimicrob Chemother. 1993;31(Suppl A):39-60.

St. Peter WL, Redic-Kill KA, Haltenson CE. Clinical pharmacokinetics of antibiotics in patients with impaired renal function. Clin Pharmacokinet. 1992;22:169-210.

Teicoplanin

Bonati M, Traina GL, Gentile MG, et al. Pharmacokinetics of intraperitoneal teicoplanin in patients with chronic renal failure on continuous ambulatory peritoneal dialysis. Br J Pharmacol. 1988;25:761-5.

Domart Y, Pierre C, Clair B, et al. Pharmacokinetics of teicoplanin in critically ill patients with varying degrees of renal impairment. Antimicrob Agents Chemother. 1987;31:1600-4.

Falcoz C, Ferry N, Pozet N, et al. Pharmacokinetics of teicoplanin in renal failure. Antimicrob Agents Chemother. 1987;31:1255-62.

Golper TA, Gleason JR, Vincent HH, et al. Drug removal during high efficiency and high flux hemodialysis. Contemp Iss Nephrol. 1993;27:175-208.

Keane WF, Everett ED, Golper TA, et al. Peritoneal dialysis-related peritonitis treatment recommendations: 1993 update. Perit Dial Int. 1993;13:14-28.

McNulty CA, Garden GM, Wise R, et al. The pharmacokinetics and tissue penetration of teicoplanin. J Antimicrob Chemother. 1985;16:743-9.

St. Peter WL, Redic-Kill KA, Haltenson CE. Clinical pharmacokinetics of antibiotics in patients with impaired renal function. Clin Pharmacokinet. 1992;22:169-210.

Trimethoprim

Golper TA, Gleason JR, Vincent HH, et al. Drug removal during high efficiency and high flux hemodialysis. Contemp Iss Nephrol. 1993;27:175-208.

Keane WF, Everett ED, Golper TA, et al. Peritoneal dialysis-related peritonitis treatment recommendations: 1993 update. Perit Dial Int. 1993;13:14-28.

Myre SA, McCann J, First MR, et al. Effect of trimethoprim on serum creatinine in healthy and chronic renal failure volunteers. Ther Drug Monit. 1987;9:161-5.

St. Peter WL, Redic-Kill KA, Haltenson CE. Clinical pharmacokinetics of antibiotics in patients with impaired renal function. Clin Pharmacokinet. 1992;22:169-210.

Vancomycin

Barth RH, DeVincenzo N. Use of vancomycin in high-flux hemodialysis: experience with 130 courses of therapy. Kidney Inter. 1996;50:929-36.

Brown DL, Manro LS. Vancomycin dosing chart for use in patients with renal impairment. Am J Kid Dis. 1988;11:15-9.

Cutler NR, Narang PK, Lesko LJ, et al. Vancomycin disposition: the importance of age. Clin Pharmacol Ther. 1984;36:803-10.

DeSoi CA, Sahm DF, Umans JG. Vancomycin elimination during high-flux hemodialysis: kinetic model and comparison of four membranes. Am J Kid Dis. 1992;20:354-60.

Golper TA, Noonan HM, Elzinga L, et al. Vancomycin pharmacokinetics: renal handling and nonrenal clearances in normal human subjects. Clin Pharmacol Ther. 1988;43:565-70.

Magere BE, Arroyo JC, Rosansly SJ, et al. Vancomycin pharmacokinetics in patients with peritonitis on peritoneal dialysis. Antimicrob Agents Chemother. 1983;23:710-4.

Moellering RC Jr, Krogstad DJ, Greenblatt DJ. Vancomycin therapy in patients with impaired renal function: a nomogram for dosage. Ann Intern Med. 1981;94:343-6.

Touchette MA, Patel RV, Anandan JV, et al. Vancomycin removal by high-flux polysulfone hemodialysis membranes in critically ill patients with end-stage renal disease. Am J Kid Dis. 1995;26:469-74.

PENICILLINS

Amoxicillin

Adam D, de Visser I, Koeppe P. Pharmacokinetics of amoxicillin and clavulanic acid administered alone and in combination. Antimicrob Agents Chemother. 1982;22:353-7.

Davies BE, Boon R, Horton R, et al. Pharmacokinetics of amoxicillin and clavulanic acid in hemodialysis patients following intravenous administration of Augmentin. Br J Clin Pharmacol. 1988;26:385-90.

Francke E, Appel GB, Neu HC. Kinetics of intravenous amoxicillin in patients on long-term dialysis. Clin Pharmacol Ther. 1979;26:31-5.

Horber FF, Frey FJ, Descoeudres C, et al. Differential effect of impaired renal function on the kinetics of clavulanic acid and amoxicillin. Antimicrob Agents Chemother. 1986;29:614-9.

Humbert G, Spyker DA, Fillastre JP, et al. Pharmacokinetics of amoxicillin: dosage nomogram for patients with impaired renal function. Antimicrob Agents Chemother. 1979;15:28-33.

Zarowny D, Ogilvie R, Tamblyn D, et al. Pharmacokinetics of amoxicillin. Clin Pharmacol Ther. 1974;16:1045-51.

Ampicillin

Jusko WJ, Lewis GP, Schmitt GW. Ampicillin and hetacillin pharmacokinetics in normal and anephric subjects. Clin Pharmacol Ther. 1973;14:90-8.

Wright N, Wise R. The elimination of sulbactam alone and combined with ampicillin in patients with renal dysfunction. Antimicrob Agents Chemother. 1967;7:767-9.

Azlocillin

Leroy A, Humbert G, Godin M, et al. Pharmacokinetics of azlocillin in subjects with normal and impaired renal function. Antimicrob Agents Chemother. 1980;17:344-9.

Whelton A, Stout RL, Delgado FA. Azlocillin kinetics during extracorporeal hemodialysis and peritoneal dialysis. J Antimicrob Chemother. 1983;11(Suppl B):89-95.

Dicloxacillin

McCloskey RV, Hayes Jr CP. Plasma levels of dicloxacillin in oliguric patients and the effect of hemodialysis. Antimicrob Agents Chemother. 1967;770-2.

Nauta EH, Mattie H. Dicloxacillin and cloxacillin: pharmacokinetics in healthy and hemodialysis subjects. Clin Pharmacol Ther. 1976;20:98-108.

Williams Jr TW, Lawson SA, Brook MI, et al. Effect of hemodialysis on dicloxacillin concentration in plasma. Antimicrob Agents Chemother. 1967;7:767-9.

Methicillin

Barza M, Weinstein L. Pharmacokinetics of the penicillins in man. Clin Pharmacokinet. 1976;1:297-308.

Bulger RJ, Lindholm DD, Murray JS, et al. Effect of uremia on methicillin and oxacillin blood levels. JAMA. 1964;187:319-22.

Mezlocillin

Aronoff GR, Sloan RS, Stanish RA, et al. Mezlocillin dose dependent elimination kinetics in renal impairment. Eur J Clin Pharmacol. 1982;21:505-9.

Kampf, D, Schurig R, Weihermuller K, et al. Effects of impaired renal function, hemodialysis, and peritoneal dialysis on the pharmacokinetics of mezlocillin. Antimicrob Agents Chemother. 1980;18:81-7.

Nafcillin

Rudnick M, Morrison G, Walker B, et al. Renal failure, hemodialysis and nafcillin kinetics. Clin Pharmacol Ther. 1976;20:413-23.

Penicillin G

No references

Penicillin VK

No references

Piperacillin

Aronoff GR, Sloan RS, Brier ME, et al. The effect of piperacillin dose on elimination kinetics in renal impairment. Eur J Clin Pharmacol. 1983;24:543-7.

Francke EL, Appel GB, Neu HC. Pharmacokinetics of intravenous piperacillin in patients undergoing chronic hemodialysis. Antimicrob Agents Chemother. 1979;16:788-91.

Ticarcillin

Parry MF, Neu HC. Pharmacokinetics of ticarcillin in patients with abnormal renal function. J Infect Dis. 1976;133:46-9.

QUINOLONE ANTIBIOTICS

Cinoxacin

Elipoulos GM. New quinolones: pharmacology, pharmacokinetics and dosing in patients with renal insufficiency. Rev Infect Dis. 1988;10(Suppl 1):S102-5.

Fillastre JP, Leroy A, Moulin B, et al. Pharmacokinetics of quinolones in renal insufficiency. J Antimicrob Chemother. 1990;26(Suppl B):51-60.

Sisca TA, Heel RC, Romankiewicz JA. Cinoxacin: a review of its pharmacological properties and therapeutic efficacy in the treatment of urinary tract infection. Drugs. 1983;25:544-69.

Wolfson JS, Hooper DC. Pharmacokinetics of quinolones: newer aspects. Eur J Clin Microbiol Infect Dis. 1991;10:267-74.

Ciprofloxacin

Aronoff GR, Kenner CH, Sloan RS, et al. Multiple-dose ciprofloxacin kinetics in normal subjects. Clin Pharmacol Ther. 1984;36:384-8.

Elipoulos GM. New quinolones: pharmacology, pharmacokinetics and dosing in patients with renal insufficiency. Rev Infect Dis. 1988;10(Suppl 1):S102-5.

Fillastre JP, Leroy A, Moulin B, et al. Pharmacokinetics of quinolones in renal insufficiency. J Antimicrob Chemother. 1990;26(Suppl B):51-60.

Forrest A, Weir M, Plaisance KI, et al. Relationship between renal function and disposition of oral ciprofloxacin. Antimicrob Agents Chemother. 1988;32:1537-40.

Golper TA, Hartstein AI, Moorthland VH, et al. Effects of antacids and dialysate dwell times on multiple dose pharmacokinetics of oral ciprofloxacin in patients on CAPD. Antimicrob Agents Chemother. 1987;31:1787-90.

Hoffken G, Lode H, Prinzing C, et al. Pharmacokinetics of ciprofloxacin after oral and parenteral administration. Antimicrob Agents Chemother. 1985;27:375-9.

Shah A, Lettieri J, Blum R, et al. Pharmacokinetics of intravenous ciprofloxacin in normal and renally impaired subjects. J Antimicrob Chemother. 1996;38:103-16.

Wolfson JS, Hooper DC. Pharmacokinetics of quinolones: newer aspects. Eur J Clin Microbiol Infect Dis. 1991;10:267-74.

Fleroxacin

Elipoulos GM. New quinolones: pharmacology, pharmacokinetics and dosing in patients with renal insufficiency. Rev Infect Dis. 1988;10(Suppl 1):S102-5.

Fillastre JP, Leroy A, Moulin B, et al. Pharmacokinetics of quinolones in renal insufficiency. J Antimicrob Chemother. 1990;26(Suppl B):51-60.

Stuck AE, Frey FJ, Heizmann O, et al. Pharmacokinetics and metabolism of intravenous and oral fleroxacin in patients on continuous ambulatory peritoneal dialysis. Antimicrob Agents Chemother. 1989;33:373-81.

Wolfson JS, Hooper DC. Pharmacokinetics of quinolones: newer aspects. Eur J Clin Microbiol Infect Dis. 1991;10:267-74.

Levofloxacin

Davis R, Bryson HM. Levofloxacin: a review of its antibacterial activity, pharmacokinetics and therapeutic efficacy. Drugs. 1994;47:677-700.

Fillastre JP, Leroy A, Moulin B, et al. Pharmacokinetics of quinolones in renal insufficiency. J Antimicrob Chemother. 1990;26(Suppl B):51-60.

Gisclon LG, Curtin CR, Chien SC, et al. The pharmacokinetics of levofloxacin in subjects with renal impairment, and in subjects receiving hemodialysis or continuous ambulatory peritoneal dialysis [Abstract]. Abstr Intersci Conf Antimicrob Agents Chemother. 1996;36:A013.

Goodwin SD, Gallis HA, Chow AT, et al. Pharmacokinetics and safety of levofloxacin in patients with human immunodeficiency virus infection. Antimicrob Agents Chemother. 1994;38:799-804.

Saito A, Oguchi K, Harada Y, et al. Pharmacokinetics of levofloxacin in patients with impaired renal function. Chemotherapy. 1992;40(Suppl 3):188-95.

Lomefloxacin

Blum RA, Schultz RW, Schentag JJ. Pharmacokinetics of lomefloxacin in renally compromised patients. Antimicrob Agents Chemother. 1990;34:2364-8.

Elipoulos GM. New quinolones: pharmacology, pharmacokinetics and dosing in patients with renal insufficiency. Rev Infect Dis. 1988;10(Suppl 1):S102-5.

Fillastre JP, Leroy A, Moulin B, et al. Pharmacokinetics of quinolones in renal insufficiency. J Antimicrob Chemother. 1990;26(Suppl B):51-60.

Leroy A, Filastre JP, Humbert G. Lomefloxacin pharmacokinetics in subjects with normal and impaired renal function. Antimicrob Agents Chemother. 1990;34:17-20.

Wolfson JS, Hooper DC. Pharmacokinetics of quinolones: newer aspects. Eur J Clin Microbiol Infect Dis. 1991;10:267-74.

Nalidixic Acid

Dash H, Mills J. Severe metabolic acidosis associated with nalidixic acid overdose [Letter]. Ann Intern Med. 1976;84:570-1.

Elipoulos GM. New quinolones: pharmacology, pharmacokinetics and dosing in patients with renal insufficiency. Rev Infect Dis. 1988;10(Suppl 1):S102-5.

Ferry N, Cuisinaud G, Pozet N, et al. Nalidixic acid kinetics after single and repeated oral doses. Clin Pharmacol Ther. 1981;29:695-8.

Fillastre JP, Leroy A, Moulin B, et al. Pharmacokinetics of quinolones in renal insufficiency. J Antimicrob Chemother. 1990;26(Suppl B):51-60.

Wolfson JS, Hooper DC. Pharmacokinetics of quinolones: newer aspects. Eur J Clin Microbiol Infect Dis. 1991;10:267-74.

Norfloxacin

Elipoulos GM. New quinolones: pharmacology, pharmacokinetics and dosing in patients with renal insufficiency. Rev Infect Dis. 1988;10(Suppl 1):S102-5.

Fillastre JP, Leroy A, Moulin B, et al. Pharmacokinetics of quinolones in renal insufficiency. J Antimicrob Chemother. 1990;26(Suppl B):51-60.

Holmes B, Brogden RN, Richards DM. Norfloxacin: a review of its antibacterial activity, pharmacokinetic properties and therapeutic use. Drugs. 1985;30:482-513.

Wolfson JS, Hooper DC. Pharmacokinetics of quinolones: newer aspects. Eur J Clin Microbiol Infect Dis. 1991;10:267-74.

Ofloxacin

Elipoulos GM. New quinolones: pharmacology, pharmacokinetics and dosing in patients with renal insufficiency. Rev Infect Dis. 1988;10(Suppl 1):S102-5.

Fillastre JP, Leroy A, Hambert G. Ofloxacin pharmacokinetics in renal failure. Antimicrob Agents Chemother. 1987;31:156-60.

Fillastre JP, Leroy A, Moulin B, et al. Pharmacokinetics of quinolones in renal insufficiency. J Antimicrob Chemother. 1990;26(Suppl B):51-60.

Lameire N, Rosenkranz B, Malercyk V, et al. Ofloxacin pharmacokinetics in chronic renal failure and dialysis. Clin Pharmacokinet. 1991;21:357-71.

Lode H, Hoffken G, Prinzing C, et al. Comparative pharmacokinetics of new quinolones. Drugs. 1987;34(Suppl 1):21-5.

White LD, MacGowan AP, Macket IG, et al. The pharmacokinetics of ofloxacin, desmethyl ofloxacin and ofloxacin *N*-oxide in hemodialysis patients with end-stage renal failure. J Antimicrob Chemother. 1988;22(Suppl C):65-72.

Wolfson JS, Hooper DC. Pharmacokinetics of quinolones: newer aspects. Eur J Clin Microbiol Infect Dis. 1991;10:267-74.

Pefloxacin

Elipoulos GM. New quinolones: pharmacology, pharmacokinetics and dosing in patients with renal insufficiency. Rev Infect Dis. 1988;10(Suppl 1):S102-5.

Fillastre JP, Leroy A, Moulin B, et al. Pharmacokinetics of quinolones in renal insufficiency. J Antimicrob Chemother. 1990;26(Suppl B):51-60.

Montay G, Jacquot C, Bariety J, et al. Pharmacokinetics of pefloxacin in renal insufficiency. Eur J Clin Pharmacol. 1985;29:345-9.

Schmit JL, Hary L, Bou P, et al. Pharmacokinetics of single dose intravenous, oral and intraperitoneal pefloxacin in patients on chronic ambulatory peritoneal dialysis. Antimicrob Agents Chemother. 1991;35:1492-4.

Wolfson JS, Hooper DC. Pharmacokinetics of quinolones: newer aspects. Eur J Clin Microbiol Infect Dis. 1991;10:267-74.

Sparfloxacin

Fillastre JP, Leroy A, Moulin B, et al. Pharmacokinetics of quinolones in renal insufficiency. J Antimicrob Chemother. 1990;26(Suppl B):51-60.

Fillastre JP, Montay G, Bruno R, et al. Pharmacokinetics of sparfloxacin in patients with renal impairment. Antimicrob Agents Chemother. 1994;38:733-7.

Montay G, Bruno R, Vergniol JC, et al. Pharmacokinetics of sparfloxacin in humans after single oral administration at doses of 200, 400, 600, and 800 mg. J Clin Pharmacol. 1994;34:1071-6.

Shamada J, Nogita T, Ishibashi Y. Clinical pharmacokinetics of sparfloxacin. Clin Pharmacokinet. 1993;25:358-69.

TETRACYCLINE ANTIBIOTICS

Doxycycline

No references

Minocycline

No references

Tetracycline

No references

ANTIFUNGAL ANTIBIOTICS

Amphotericin B

Block ER, Bennett JE, Livoti LG, et al. Flucytosine and amphotericin B: hemodialysis effects on the plasma concentration and clearance: studies in man. Ann Intern Med. 1974;80:613-7.

Morgan DJ, Ching MS, Raymond K, et al. Elimination of amphotericin B in impaired renal function. Clin Pharmacol Ther. 1983;34:248-53.

Muther RS, Bennett WM. Peritoneal clearance of amphotericin B and 5-fluorocytosine. West J Med. 1980;133:157-60.

Amphotericin B Colloidal Dispersion

Amantea MA, Bowden RA, Forrest A, et al. Population pharmacokinetics and renal function-sparing effects of amphotericin B colloidal dispersion in patients receiving bone marrow transplants. Antimicrob Agents Chemother. 1995;39:2042-7.

Sanders SW, Buchi KN, Goddard MS, et al. Single-dose pharmacokinetics and tolerance of a cholesterol sulfate complex of amphotericin B administered to healthy volunteers. Antimicrob Agents Chemother. 1991;35:1029-34.

Amphotericin B Lipid Complex

Humphreys H, Oliver DA, Winter R, et al. Liposomal amphotericin B and continuous venous-venous haemofiltration [Letter]. J Antimicrob Chemother. 1994; 33:1070-1.

Kan VL, Bennett JE, Amantea MA, et al. Comparative safety, tolerance, and pharmacokinetics of amphotericin B lipid complex and amphotericin B desoxycholate in healthy male volunteers. J Infect Dis. 1991;164:418-421.

Tomlin M, Priestley GS. Elimination of liposomal amphotericin by hemodiafiltration [Letter]. Intensive Care Med. 1995;21:699-700.

Fluconazole

Berl T, Wilner KD, Gardner M, et al. Pharmacokinetics of fluconazole in renal failure. J Am Soc Nephrol. 1995;2:242-7.

Thomas MG, Ellis-Pegler RB. Fluconazole treatment of *Candida glabrata* peritonitis. J Antimicrob Chemother. 1989;24:94-5.

Flucytosine

Cutler RE, Blair AD, Kelly MR. Flucytosine kinetics in subjects with normal and impaired renal function. Clin Pharmacol Ther. 1978;24:333-42.

Griseofulvin

No references

Itraconazole

Boelaert J, Schurgers M, Matthys E, et al. Itraconazole pharmacokinetics in patients with renal dysfunction. Antimicrob Agents Chemother. 1988;32:1595-7.

Hardin TC, Graybill JR, Fetchick R, et al. Pharmacokinetics of itraconazole following oral administration to normal volunteers. Antimicrob Agents Chemother. 1988;32:1310-3.

Heykants J, Van Peer A, Van de Vilde V, et al. Clinical pharmacokinetics of itraconazole: a review. Mycoses. 1989;32(Suppl 1):67-87.

Ketoconazole

Daneshmend TK, Warnock DW, Turner A, et al. Pharmacokinetics of ketoconazole in normal subjects. J Antimicrob Chemother. 1981;8:299-304.

Heel RC, Brogden RN, Carmine A, et al. Ketoconazole: a review of its therapeutic efficacy in superficial and systemic fungal infections. Drugs. 1982;23:1-36.

Johnson RJ, Blair AD, Ahmad S. Ketoconazole kinetics in chronic peritoneal dialysis. Clin Pharmacol Ther. 1985;37:325-9.

Miconazole

Lewis PJ, Boelaert J, Daneels R. Pharmacokinetic profile of intravenous miconazole in man: comparison of normal subjects and patients with renal insufficiency. Eur J Clin Pharmacol. 1976;10:49-54.

ANTIMYCOBACTERIAL ANTIBIOTICS

Capreomycin

Lehmann CR, Garrett LE, Winn RE, et al. Capreomycin kinetics in renal impairment and clearance by hemodialysis. Am Rev Respir Dis. 1988;138:1312-3.

Cycloserine

No references

Ethambutol

Lee CS, Marbury TC, Benet LZ. Clearance calculations in hemodialysis: application to blood, plasma, and dialysate measurements for ethambutol. J Pharmacokinet Biopharm. 1980;8:69-81.

Varughese A, Brater DC, Benet LZ, et al. Ethambutol kinetics in patients with impaired renal function. Am Rev Resp Dis. 1986;134:34-8.

Ethionamide

No references

Isoniazid

Gold CH, Buchanan N, Tringham V, et al. Isoniazid pharmacokinetics in patients with chronic renal failure. Clin Nephrol. 1976;6:365-9.

PAS

No references

Pyrazinimide

Lacroix C, Hermelin A, Guiberteau R, et al. Haemodialysis of pyrazinimide in uraemic patients. Eur J Clin Pharmacol. 1989;37:309-11.

Stamatakis G, Montes C, Trouvin JH, et al. Pyrazinimide and pyrazinoic acid pharmacokinetics in patients with chronic renal failure. Clin Nephrol. 1988;30:230-4.

Woo J, Leung A, Chan K, et al. Pyrazinimide and rifampin regimens for patients on maintenance dialysis. Int J Artif Organs. 1988;11:181-5.

ANTIPARASITIC ANTIBIOTICS

Atovaquone

Dixon R, Pozniak AL, Watt HM, et al. Single-dose and steady-state pharmacokinetics of a novel microfluidized suspension of atovaquone in human immunodeficiency virus-seropositive patients. Antimicrob Agents Chemother. 1996;40:556-60.

Hughes WT, Kennedy W, Shenep JL, et al. Safety and pharmacokinetics of 566C80, a hydroxynaphthoquinone with anti-*Pneumocystis carinii* activity: a phase I study in human immunodeficiency virus (HIV)-infected men. J Infect Dis. 1991;163:843-8.

Chloroquine

Gustafsson LL, Walker O, Alvan G, et al. Disposition of chloroquine in man after single intravenous and oral doses. Br J Clin Pharmacol. 1983;15:471-9.

Mefloquine

Crevoisier CA, Joseph I, Fischer M, et al. Influence of hemodialysis on plasma concentration-time profiles of mefloquine in two patients with end-stage renal disease:

a prophylactic drug monitoring study. Antimicrob Agents Chemother. 1995;39:1892-5.

Pentamidine

Conte JE Jr. Pharmacokinetics of intravenous pentamidine in patients with normal renal function or receiving hemodialysis. J Infect Dis. 1991;163:169-75.
Conte JE Jr, Upton RA, Lin ET. Pentamidine pharmacokinetics in patients with AIDS with impaired renal function. J Infect Dis. 1987;156:885-90.

Primaquine

Greaves J, Evans DAP, Gilles HM, et al. Plasma kinetics and urinary excretion of primaquine in man. Br J Clin Pharmacol. 1980;10:399-405.
Mihaly GW, Ward SA, Edwards G, et al. Pharmacokinetics of primaquine in man: identification of the carboxylic acid derivative as a major plasma metabolite. Br J Clin Pharmacol. 1984;17:441-6.

Pyrimethamine

No references

Quinine

Davies JG, Greenwood EF, Kingswood JC, et al. Quinine clearance in continuous venovenous hemofiltration. Ann Pharmacother. 1996;30:487-90.
Krishna S, White NJ. Pharmacokinetics of quinine, chloroquine and amodiaquine. Clinical implications. Clin Pharmacokinet. 1996;30:263-99.
Rimchala P, Karlbwang J, Sukontason K, et al. Pharmacokinetics of quinine in patients with chronic renal failure. Eur J Clin Pharmacol. 1996;49:497-501.

Trimetrexate

Ho DHW, Covington WP, Legha SS, et al. Clinical pharmacology of trimetrexate. Clin Pharmacol Ther. 1987;42:351-6.
Marshall JL, DeLap RJ. Clinical pharmacokinetics and pharmacology of trimetrexate. Clin Pharmacokinet. 1994;26:190-200.

ANTITUBERCULOUS ANTIBIOTICS

Rifampin

Acocella, G. Clinical pharmacokinetics of rifampin. Clin Pharmacokinet. 1978;3:108-27.
Kenny MT, Strates B. Metabolism and pharmacokinetics of the antibiotic rifampin. Drug Metab Rev. 1981;12:159-218.

ANTIVIRAL AGENTS

Acyclovir

Krasny HC, Liao S, Demiranda P, et al. Influence of hemodialysis on acyclovir pharmacokinetics in patients with chronic renal failure. Am J Med. 1982;73:202-4.

Laskin OL. Clinical pharmacokinetics of acyclovir. Clin Pharmacokinet. 1983;8:187-201.

Amantadine

Horadam VW, Sharp JG, Smilack JD, et al. Pharmacokinetics of amantadine hydrochloride in subjects with normal and impaired renal function. Ann Intern Med. 1981;94:454-8.

Wu MJ, Ing TS, Soung LS, et al. Amantadine hydrochloride pharmacokinetics in patients with impaired renal function. Clin Nephrol. 1982;17:19-23.

Cidofovir

Cundy KC, Petty BG, Flaherty J, et al. Clinical pharmacokinetics of cidofovir in human immunodeficiency virus-infected patients. Antimicrob Agents Chemother. 1995;39:1247-52.

Lalezari JP, Drew WL, Glutzer E, et al. (S)-1-[3-hydroxy-2-(phosphonyl-methoxy)propyl]cytosine (Cidofovir): results of aphase I/II study of a novel antiviral nucleotide analog. J Infect Dis. 1995;171:788-96.

Delavirdine

No references

Didanosine

Hartman NR, Yarchoan R, Pluda JM, et al. Pharmacokinetics of 2´,3´-dideoxy-adenosine and 2´-3´-dideoxyinosine in patients with severe human immunodeficiency virus infection. Clin Pharmacol Ther. 1990;47:647-54.

Knupp CA, Shyu WC, Dolin R, et al. Pharmacokinetics of didanosine in patients with acquired immunodeficiency syndrome or acquired immunodeficiency-related complex. Clin Pharmacol Ther. 1991;49:523-35.

Singlas E, Taburet AM, Lebas FB, et al. Didanosine pharmacokinetics in patients with normal and impaired renal function: influence of hemodialysis. Antimicrob Agents Chemother. 1992;36:1519-24.

Famciclovir

Boike SC, Pue MA, Freed MI, et al. Pharmacokinetics of famciclovir in subjects with varying degrees of renal impairment. Clin Pharmacol Ther. 1994;55:418-26.

Pue MA, Benet LZ. Pharmacokinetcs of famciclovir in man. Antiviral Chem Chemother. 1993;4(Suppl 1):47-55.

Foscarnet

Alexander AC, Akers A, Matzke GR. Disposition of foscarnet during peritoneal dialysis. Ann Pharmacother. 1996;30:1106-9.

Aweeka FT, Pirrung D, Lizak P, et al. Pharmacokinetics of foscarnet in patients with varying degrees of renal function and hemodialysis [Abstract]. Clin Pharmacol Ther. 1994;55:195.

MacGregor RR, Graziani AL, Weiss R, et al. Successful foscarnet therapy for cytomegalovirus retinitis in an AIDS patient undergoing hemodialysis: rationale for empiric dosing and plasma level monitoring. J Infect Dis. 1991;164:785-7.

Ganciclovir

Fletcher C, Sawchuk R, Chinnock MT, et al. Human pharmacokinetics of the antiviral drug DHPG. Clin Pharmacol Ther. 1986;40:281-6.

Jackson MA, DeMiranda P, Cederberg DM, et al. Human pharmacokinetics and tolerance of oral ganciclovir. Antimicrob Agents Chemother. 1987;31:1251-4.

Lake KD, Fletcher CV, Love KR, et al. Ganciclovir pharmacokinetics during renal impairment. Antimicrob Agents Chemother. 1988;32:1899-900.

Sommadossi J, Bevan R, Ling T, et al. Clinical pharmacokinetics of ganciclovir in patients with normal and impaired renal function. Rev Infect Dis. 1988;10 (Suppl 3): 507.

Swan SK, Munar MY, Wigger MA, et al. Pharmacokinetics of ganciclovir in a patient undergoing hemodialysis. Am J Kidney Dis. 1991;17:69-72.

Ganciclovir (Oral)

Anderson RD, Griffy KG, Jung D, et al. Ganciclovir absolute bioavailablity and steady-state pharmacokinetics after oral administration of two 3000 mg/d dosing regimens in human immunodeficiency virus-and cytomegalovirus-seropositive patients. Clin Therapeutics. 1995;17:425-32.

Indinavir

Balani SK, Woolf EJ, Hoagland VL, et al. Disposition of indinavir, a potent HIV-1 protease inhibitor, after an oral dose in humans. Drug Metab Dispos. 1996;24:1389-94.

Lamivudine

Heald AE, Hsyu PH, Yuen GJ, et al. Pharmacokinetcs of lamivudine in human immunodeficiency virus-infected patients with renal dysfunction. Anitmicrob Agents Chemother. 1996;40:1514-9.

Yuen GJ, Morris DM, Mydlow PK, et al. Pharmacokinetics, absolute bioavailability, and absorption characteristics of lamivudine. J Clin Pharmacol. 1995;35:1174-80.

Nelfinavir

No references

Nevirapine

Cheeseman SH, Hattox SE, McLaughlin MM, et al. Pharmacokinetics of nevirapine: initial single-rising-dose study in humans. Antimicrob Agents Chemother. 1993;37:178-82.

Havlir D, Cheeseman SH, McLaughlin M, et al. High-dose nevirapine: safety, pharmacokinetics, and antiviral effect in patients with human immunodeficiency virus infection. J Infect Dis. 1995;171:537-45.

Ribavirin

Kramer TH, Gaar GG, Ray CG, et al. Hemodialysis clearance of intravenously administered ribavirin. Antimicrob Agents Chemother. 1990;34:489-90.

Laskin OL, Longstreth JA, Hart CC, et al. Ribavirin disposition in high risk patients for acquired immunodeficiency syndrome. Clin Pharmacol Ther. 1987;41:546-55.

Lertora JJ, Rege AB, La Cour JT, et al. Pharmacokinetics and long term tolerance to ribavirin in asymptomatic patients infected with immunodeficiency virus. Clin Pharmacol Ther. 1991;50:442-9.

Paroni R, Del Puppo M, Borght C, et al. Pharmacokinetics of ribavirin and urinary excretion of the major metabolite 1,2,4-triazole-3-carboxamide in normal volunteers. Int J Clin Pharmacol Ther Toxicol. 1989;27:302-7.

Roberts RB, Laskin OL, Laurence J, et al. Ribavirin pharmacodynamics in high risk patients for acquired immunodeficiency syndrome. Clin Pharmacol Ther. 1987;42:365-73.

Rifabutin

Narang PK, Schoenfelder J, Bianchine JR. Impact of altered rifabutin disposition in renal disease on its safety in AIDS patients. AIDS. 1992;6(Suppl 1):90.

Skinner MH, Hsieh M, Torseth J, et al. Pharmacokinetics of rifabutin. Antimicrob Agents Chemother. 1989;33:1237-41.

Ritonavir

Danner SA, Carr A, Leonard JM, et al. A short-term study of the safety, pharmacokinetics, and efficacy of ritonavir, an inhibitor of HIV-1 protease. New Engl J Med. 1995;333:1528-33.

Hsu A, Granneman DR, Witt G, et al. Multiple-dose pharmacokinetics of ritonavir in human immunodeficiency virus-infected subjects. Antimicrob Agents Chemother. 1997;4:898-905.

Markowitz M, Saag M, Powderly WG, et al. A preliminary study of ritonavir, an inhibitor of HIV-1 protease, to treat HIV-1 infection. New Engl J Med. 1995;333:1534-9.

Saquinavir

No references

Stavudine

Dudley MN, Graham KK, Kaul S, et al. Pharmacokinetics of stavudine in patients with AIDS or AIDS-related complex. J Infect Dis. 1992;166:480-5.

Horton CM, Dudley MN, Kaul S, et al. Population pharmacokinetics of stavudine (d4T) in patients with AIDS or advanced AIDS-related complex. Antimicrob Agents Chemother. 1995;39:2309-15.

Valacyclovir

Soul-Lawton J, Seaber E, On N, et al. Absolute bioavailability and metabolic disposition of valaciclovir, the L-valylester of acyclovir, following oral administration of humans. Antimicrob Agents Chemother. 1995;39:2759-64.

Weller S, Blum MR, Doucette M, et al. Pharmacokinetics of the acyclovir pro-drug valaciclovir after escalating single- and multiple-dose administration to normal volunteers. Clin Pharmacol Ther. 1993;54:595-605.

Vidarabine

Aronoff GR, Szwed JJ, Nelson RL, et al. Hypoxanthine-arabinoside pharmacokinetics after adenine arabinoside administration to a patient with renal failure. Antimicrob Agents Chemother. 1980;18:212-4.

Zalcitabine

Gustavson LE, Fukuda EK, Rubio FA, et al. A pilot study of the bioavailability and pharmacokinetics of 2´,3´-dideoxycytidine in patients with AIDS or AIDS-related complex. J Acquir Immune Defic Syndr. 1990;3:28-31.

Klecker RW, Collins JM, Yarchoan RC, et al. Pharmacokinetics of 2´,3´-dideoxycytidine in patients with AIDS and related disorders. J Clin Pharmacol. 1988;28:837-42.

Zidovudine

Gallicano KD, Tobe S, Saha J, et al. Pharmacokinetics of single and chronic dose zidovudine in two HIV+ patients undergoing CAPD. J Acquir Immune Defic Syndr. 1992;5:242-50.

Gleason J, Brier ME. Zidovudine: therapeutic recommendations for its use in renal failure. Semin Dialysis. 1990;3:101-4.

Klecker RW, Collins JM, Vorchoan R, et al. Plasma and CSF pharmacokinetics of 3-azido-3-deoxy-thymidine: a novel pyrimidine analog with potential application for treatment of patients with AIDS and related diseases. Clin Pharmacol Ther. 1987;41:407-12.

Kremer D, Munar MY, Kohlhepp SJ, et al. Zidovudine pharmacokinetics in five HIV seronegative patients undergoing continuous ambulatory peritoneal dialysis. Pharmacotherapy. 1992;12:56-60.

Singlas E, Pioger JC, Taburet AM, et al. Zidovudine disposition in patients with severe renal impairment: influence of hemodialysis. Clin Pharmacol Ther. 1989;46:190-7.

Miscellaneous Agents

ANTICOAGULANTS

Alteplase (Tissue-Type Plasminogen Activator [tPa])

No references

Anistreplase

No references

Dipyridamole

Fitzgerald GA. Dipyridamole. N Engl J Med. 1987;316:1247-51.

Mahoney G, Wolfram KM, Cochetto D, et al. Dipyridamole kinetics. Clin Pharmacol Ther. 1982;31:330-8.

Heparin

Kandrotas RJ. Heparin pharmacokinetics and pharmacodynamics. Clin Pharmacokinet. 1992;22:359-74.

Perry PJ, Herron GR, King JC. Heparin half-life in normal and impaired renal function. Clin Pharmacol Ther. 1974;16:514-9.

Thien AN, Bjornsson J. Heparin elimination in uraemic patients on hemodialysis. Scand J Haematol. 1977;17:29-35.

Iloprost

Hildebrand M. Pharmacokinetics of iloprost in patients with chronic renal failure on hemodialysis. Int J Clin Pharm Res. 1990;10:285-92.

Indobufen

Savazzi GM, Castiglioni A, Cavatorta A. Effect of renal insufficiency on the pharmacokinetics of indobufen. Curr Therap Res. 1984;36:119-25.

Wiseman LR, Fitton A, Buckley MM. Indobufen. Drugs. 1992;44:445-64.

Low-Molecular-Weight Heparin

Weitz JI. Low-molecular-weight heparins. N Engl J Med. 1997;337:688-98.

Streptokinase

Grierson DS, Bjornsson TD. Pharmacokinetics of streptokinase in patients based on amidolytic activator complex activity. Clin Pharmacol Ther. 1987;41:304-13.

Sulfinpyrazone

Margulies EH, White AM, Sherry S. Sulfinpyrazone: a review of its pharmacological properties and therapeutic use. Drugs. 1980;20:179-97.

Pedersen AK, Jakobsen P, Kampmann JP, et al. Clinical pharmacokinetics and potentially important drug interactions of sulfinpyrazone. Clin Pharmacokinet. 1982;7:42-56.

Sulotroban

No references

Ticlopidine

Kelly JG, O'Malley K. Clinical pharmacokinetics of oral anticoagulants. Clin Pharmacokinet. 1979;4:1-15.

Saltiel E, Ward A. Ticlopidine: a review of its pharmacodynamic and pharmacokinetics properties, and therapeutic efficacy in platelet-dependent disease states. Drugs. 1987;34:222-62.

Van Peer A, Belparie F, Bogaert M. Warfarin elimination and responsiveness in patients with renal dysfunction. J Clin Pharmacol. 1978;18:84-8.

Tranexamic Acid

Astedt B. Clinical pharmacology of tranexamic acid. Scand J Gastroenterol Suppl. 1987;137:22-5.

Pillbrant A, Schannong M, Vessman J. Pharmacokinetics and bioavailability of tranexamic acid. Eur J Clin Pharmacol. 1981;20:65-72.

Urokinase

No references

Warfarin

No references

ANTICONVULSANTS

Carbamazepine

Bertilsson L, Tomson T. Clinical pharmacokinetics and pharmacological effects of carbamazepine and carbamazepine-10,11-epoxide: an update. Clin Pharmacokinet. 1986;11:177-98.

Lee CS, Wang LH, Marbury TC, et al. Hemodialysis clearance and total body elimination of carbamazepine during chronic hemodialysis. Clin Toxicol. 1980;17:429-38.

Ethosuximide

Marbury TC, Lee CS, Perchalski RJ, et al. Hemodialysis clearance of ethosuximide in patients with chronic renal disease. Am J Hosp Pharm. 1981;38:1757-60.

Gabapentin

Bialer M. Comparative pharmacokinetics of the newer antiepileptic drugs. Clin Pharmacokinet. 1993;24:441-52.

Lamotrigine

Cohen AF, Land GS, Breimer DD, et al. Lamotrigine, a new anticonvulsant: pharmacokinetics in normal humans. Clin Pharmacol Ther. 1987;42:535-41.

Rambeck B, Wolf P. Lamotrigine clinical pharmacokinetics. Clin Pharmacokinet. 1993;25:433-43.

Oxcarbazepine

No references

Phenytoin

Borga O, Hoppel C, Odar-Cederlof I, et al. Plasma levels and renal excretion of phenytoin and its metabolites in patients with renal failure. Clin Pharmacol Ther. 1979;26:306-14.

Primidone

Lee CS, Marbury TC, Perchalski RT, et al. Pharmacokinetics of primidone elimination by uremic patients. J Clin Pharmacol. 1982;22:301-8.

Sodium Valproate

Browne TR. Valproic acid. N Engl J Med. 1980;302:661-6.

Zaccara G, Messori A, Moroni F. Clinical pharmacokinetics of valproic acid—1988. Clin Pharmacokinet. 1988;15:367-89.

Topiramate

Gisclon LG, Riffits JM, Sica DA, et al. The pharmacokinetics of topiramate in subjects with renal impairment as compared to matched subjects with normal renal function. Pharm Res. 1993;10:S397.

Trimethadione

No references

Vigabatrin

Haegele KD, Huebert ND, Ebel M, et al. Pharmacokinetics of vigabatrin: implications of creatinine clearance. Clin Pharm Ther. 1988;44:558-65.

Schechter PJ. Clinical pharmacology of vigabatrin. Br J Clin Pharmacol. 1989;27:19S-22S.

ANTIHISTAMINES

H_1 ANTAGONISTS

Acrivastine

Brogden RN, McTavish D. Acrivastine. Drugs. 1991;41:927-40.

Astemizole

Richards DM, Brogden RN, Heel RC, et al. Astemizole: a review of its pharmacodynamic properties and therapeutic efficacy. Drugs. 1984;28:38-61.

Brompheniramine

No references

Cetirizine

Awni W, Yeh J, Halstenson CE, et al. Effects of hemodialysis on the pharmacokinetics of cetirizine. Eur J Clin Pharm. 1990;38:67-9.

Chlorpheniramine

No references

Diphenhydramine

No references

Erbastine

Wiseman LR, Faulds D. Erbastine. Drugs. 1996;51:260-77.

Fexofenadine

[Anonymous.] Fexofenadine. Med Lett Drugs Ther. 1996;38(986):95-6.

Flunarizine

Holmes B, Brogden RN, Heel RC, et al. Flunarizine: a review of its pharmacodynamic and pharmacokinetic properties and therapeutic use. Drugs. 1984;27:6-44.

Hydroxyzine

No references

Orphenadrine

No references

Oxatomide

Richards DM, Brogden RN, Heel RC, et al. Oxatomide: a review of its pharmacodynamic properties and therapeutic efficacy. Drugs. 1984;27:210-31.

Promethazine

No references

Terfenadine

Sorkin EM, Heel RC. Terfenadine: a review of its pharmacodynamic properties and therapeutic efficacy. Drugs. 1985;29:34-56.

Tripelennamine

No references

Triprolidine

No references

H_2 ANTAGONISTS

Cimetidine

Larsson R, Norlander B, Bodemar G, et al. Steady-state kinetics and dosage requirements of cimetidine in renal failure. Clin Pharmacokinet. 1981;6:316-25.
Somogyi A, Gugler R. Clinical pharmacokinetics of cimetidine. Clin Pharmacokinet. 1983;8:463-95.

Famotidine

Campoli-Richards DM, Clissold SP. Famotidine: pharmacodynamic and pharmacokinetic properties and a preliminary review of its therapeutic use in peptic ulcer disease and Zollinger-Ellison syndrome. Drugs. 1986;32:197-221.

Nizatidine

Price AH, Brogden RN. Nizatidine: a preliminary review of its pharmacodynamic and pharmacokinetic properties, and its therapeutic use in peptic ulcer disease. Drugs. 1988;36:521-39.

Ranitidine

Grant SM, Langtry HD, Brogden RN. Ranitidine: an updated review of its pharmacodynamic and pharmacokinetic properties and therapeutic use in peptic ulcer disease and other allied diseases. Drugs. 1989;37:801-70.

Meffin PJ, Grgurinovich N, Brooks PM, et al. Ranitidine disposition in patients with renal impairment. Br J Clin Pharmacol. 1983;16:731-4.

ANTINEOPLASTIC AGENTS

Altretamine

Damia G, D'Incalci M. Clinical pharmacokinetics of altretamine. Clin Pharmacokinet. 1995;28:439-48.

Lee CR, Faulds D. Altretamine: a review of its pharmacodynamic and pharmacokinetic properties, and therapeutic potential in cancer chemotherapy. Drugs. 1995;49:932-53.

Azathioprine

Bach JF, Dardenne M. The metabolism of azathioprine in renal failure. Transplantation. 1971;12:253-9.

Bleomycin

Bennett JM, Reich SD. Bleomycin. Ann Intern Med. 1979;90:945-8.

Dalgleish AG, Woods RL, Levi JA. Bleomycin pulmonary toxicity: its relationship to renal dysfunction. Med Pediatr Oncol. 1984;12:313-7.

Busulfan

Ehrsson H, Hassan M, Ehrnebo M, et al. Busulfan kinetics. Clin Pharmacol Ther. 1983;34:86-9.

Millard RJ. Busulfan haemorrhagic cystitis. Br J Urol. 1978;50:210-6.

Carboplatin

Calvert H, Judson I, van der Vijgh WJF. Platinum complexes in cancer medicine: pharmacokinetics and pharmacodynamics in relation to toxicity and therapeutic activity. Cancer Surv. 1993;17:189-217.

Chatelut E, Rostaing L, Gualano V, et al. Pharmacokinetics of carboplatin in a patient suffering from advanced ovarian carcinoma with hemodialysis-dependent renal insufficiency. Nephron. 1994;66:157-61.

Carmustine

Black DJ, Livingston RB. Antineoplastic drugs in 1990. Drugs. 1990;39(4): 489-501.

Muggia FM, Von Hoff DD. In: Avery's Drug Treatment. 4th ed. Speight TM, Holford N, eds. Auckland: ADIS International Limited Year. 1997, p. 1255.

Chlorambucil

Black DJ, Livingston RB. Antineoplastic drugs in 1990. Drugs. 1990;39(4): 489-501.

Cisplatin

Benisovich VI, Silverman L, Slifkin R, et al. Cisplatin-based chemotherapy in renal transplant recipients: a case report and a review of the literature. Cancer. 1996;77:160-3.

Blanchley JD, Hill JB. Renal and electrolyte disturbances associated with cisplatin. Ann Intern Med. 1981;95:628-32.

Gormley PE, Bull JM, Leroy AF, et al. Kinetics of *cis*-dichlorodiammineplatinum. Clin Pharmacol Ther. 1979;25:351-7.

Cladribine

Bryson HM, Sorkin EM. Cladribine: a review of its pharmacodynamic and pharmaco-kinetic properties and therapeutic potential in haematological malignancies. Drugs. 1993;46:872-94.

Cyclophosphamide

Lind MJ, Ardiet C. Pharmacokinetics of alkylating agents. Cancer Surv. 1993;17:157-88.

Moore MJ. Clinical pharmacokinetics of cyclophosphamide. Clin Pharmacokinet. 1991;20:194-208.

Cytarabine

Wan SH, Huffman DH, Azarnoff DL, et al. Pharmacokinetics of 1-beta-D-arabinofu-ranosylcytosine in humans. Cancer Res. 1974;34:392-7.

Daunorubicin

[Anonymous.] Drugs of choice for cancer chemotherapy. Medical Letter. 1996;39(996):21-8.

Muggia FM, Von Hoff DD. In: Avery's Drug Treatment. 4th ed. Speight TM, Holford N, eds. Auckland: ADIS International Limited Year. 1997, p. 1256.

Doxorubicin

Benjamin RS, Riggs CE Jr, Bacher NR. Plasma pharmacokinetics of adriamycin and its metabolites in humans with normal hepatic and renal function. Cancer Res. 1977;37:1416-20.

Goto M, Yoshida H, Honda A, et al. Delayed disposition of adriamycin and its active metabolite in haemodialysis patients. Eur J Clin Pharmacol. 1993;44:301-2.

Robert J, Gianni L. Pharmacokinetics and metabolism of anthracyclines. Cancer Surv. 1993;17:219-52.

Speth PA, Van Hoesel QG, Haanen C. Clinical pharmacokinetics of doxorubicin. Clin Pharmacokinet. 1988;15:15-31.

Yoshida H, Goto M, Honda A, et al. Pharmacokinetics of doxorubicin and its active metabolite in patients with normal renal function and in patients on hemodialysis. Cancer Chemother Pharmacol. 1994;33:450-4.

Epirubicin

Plosker GL, Faulds D. Epirubicin: a review of its pharmacodynamic and pharmaco-kinetic properties, and therapuetic use in cancer chemotherapy. Drugs. 1993;45:788-856.

Robert J. Clinical pharmacokinetics of epirubicin. Clin Pharmacokinet. 1994;26:428-38.

Etoposide

Clark PI, Slevin ML. The clinical pharmacology of etoposide and teniposide. Clin Pharmacokinet. 1987;12:223-52.

McLeod HL, Evans WE. Clinical pharmacokinetics and pharmacodynamics of epipodophyllotoxins. Cancer Surv. 1993;17:253-68.

Sinkule JA. Etoposide: a semisynthetic epipodophyllotoxin. Chemistry, pharmacology, pharmacokinetics, adverse effects and use as an antineoplastic agent. Pharmacotherapy. 1984;4:61-73.

Stewart CF. Use of etoposide in patients with organ dysfunction: pharmacokinetic and pharmacodynamic considerations. Cancer Chemother Pharmacol. 1994;34:S76-S83.

Fludarabine

Ross SR, McTavish D, Faulds D. Fludarabine: a review of its pharmacological proper-ties and therapeutic potential in malignancy. Drugs. 1993;45:737-59.

Fluorouracil

Diasio RB, Harris BE. Clinical pharmacology of 5-fluorouracil. Clin Pharmacokinet. 1989;16:215-37.

MacMillan WE, Wolberg WH, Welling PG. Pharmacokinetics of fluorouracil in humans. Cancer Res. 1978;38:3479-82.

Flutamide

Brogden RN, Clissold SP. Flutamide: a preliminary review of its pharmacodynamic and pharmacokinetic properties, and therapeutic efficacy in advanced prostatic can-cer. Drugs. 1989;38:185-203.

Goldspiel BR, Kohler DR. Flutamide: an antiandrogen for advanced prostate cancer. Ann Pharmacother. 1990;24:616-23.

Hydroxyurea

[Anonymous.] Drugs of choice for cancer chemotherapy. Medical Letter. 1996;39(996):21-8.

Muggia FM, Von Hoff DD. In: Avery's Drug Treatment. 4th ed. Speight TM, Holford N, eds. Auckland: ADIS International Limited. 1997;1255.

Idarubicin

Hollingshead LM, Faulds D. Idarubicin: a review of its pharmacodynamic and pharmacokinetic properties, and therapeutic potential in the chemotherapy of cancer. Drugs. 1991;42:690-719.

Robert J. Clinical pharmacokinetics of idarubicin. Clin Pharmacokinet. 1993;24:275-88.

Ifosfamide

Wagner T. Ifosfamide clinical pharmacokinetics. Clin Pharmacokinet. 1994;26:439-56.

Melphalan

Alberts DS, Chang SY, Chen HG, et al. Kinetics of intravenous melphalan. Clin Pharmacol Ther. 1979;26:73-80.

Kergueris MF, Milpied N, Moreau P, et al. Pharmacokinetics of high-dose melphalan in adults: influence of renal function. Anticancer Res. 1994;14:2379-82.

Methotrexate

Jolivet J, Cowan KH, Curt GA, et al. The pharmacology and clinical use of methotrexate. N Engl J Med. 1983;309:1094-104.

Shen DD, Azarnoff DL. Clinical pharmacokinetics of methotrexate. Clin Pharmacokinet. 1978;3:1-13.

Thomson AH, Daly M, Knepil J, et al. Methotrexate removal during haemodialysis in a patient with advanced laryngeal carcinoma. Cancer Chemother Pharmacol. 1996;38:566-70.

Mitomycin C

Den Hartigh J, McVie JG, Van Oort WS, et al. Pharmacokinetics of mitomycin C in humans. Cancer Res. 1983;43:5017-21.

Giroux L, Bettez P, Giroux L. Mitomycin C nephrotoxicity: a clinicopathologic study of 17 cases. Am J Kid Dis. 1985;6:28-39.

Mitoxantrone

Ehninger G, Schuler U, Proksch B, et al. Pharmacokinetics and metabolism of mitoxantrone: a review. Clin Pharmacokinet. 1990;18:365-80.

Faulds D, Balfour JA, Chrisp P, et al. Mitoxantrone: a review of its pharmacodynamic and pharmacokinetic properties, and therapeutic potential in the chemotherapy of cancer. Drugs. 1991;41:400-49.

Nitrosoureas

Ellis ME, Weiss RB, Kupermine M. Nephrotoxicity of lomustine: a case report and literature review. Cancer Chemother Pharmacol. 1985;15:174-5.
Oloverio VT. Toxicology and pharmacology of the nitrosoureas. Cancer Chemother Rep. 1973;4:13-20.

Paclitaxel

Dreicer R, Gustin DM, See WA, et al. Paclitaxel in advanced urothelial carcinoma: its role in patients with renal insufficiency and as salvage therapy. J Urol. 1996;156:1606-8.
Kearns CM, Gianni L, Egorin MJ. Paclitaxel pharmacokinetics and pharmacodynamics. Semin Oncol. 1995;22:16-23.
Sonnichsen DS, Relling MV. Clinical pharmacokinetics of paclitaxel. Clin Pharmacokinet. 1994;27:256-69.

Plicamycin

Kennedy BJ. Metabolic and toxic effects of mithramycin during tumor therapy. Am J Med. 1970;49:494-503.

Streptozocin

Hall-Craggs M, Brenner DE, Vigorito RD, et al. Acute renal failure and renal tubular squamous metaplasia following treatment with streptozocin. Hum Pathol. 1982;13:597-601.

Tamoxifen

Buckley MM, Goa KL. Tamoxifen: a reappraisal of its pharmacodynamic and pharmacokinetic properties, and therapeutic use. Drugs. 1989;37:451-90.

Teniposide

Clark PI, Slevin ML. The clinical pharmacology of etoposide and teniposide. Clin Pharmacokinet. 1987;12:223-52.
Sinkule JA. Etoposide: a semisynthetic epipodophyllotoxin. Chemistry, pharmacology, pharmacokinetics, adverse effects and use as an antineoplastic agent. Pharmacotherapy. 1984;4:61-73.

Topotecan

Herben VMM, ten Bokkel Huinink WW, et al. Clinical pharmacokinetics of topotecan. Clin Pharmacokinet. 1996;31:85-102.

Vinblastine

Owellen RJ, Root MA, Hains FO. Pharmacokinetics and metabolism of vinblastine in humans. Cancer Res. 1977;37:2597-602.
Rahmani R, Zhou XJ. Pharmacokinetics and metabolism of vinca alkaloids. Cancer Surv. 1993;17:269-81.

Vincristine

Owellen RJ, Root MA, Hains FO. Pharmacokinetics of vinblastine and vincristine in humans. Cancer Res. 1977;37:2603-7.

Vinorelbine

Leveque D, Jehl F. Clinical pharmacokinetics of vinorelbine. Clin Pharmacokinet. 1996;31:184-97.

ANTIPARKINSON AGENTS

Carbidopa

No references

Levodopa

Nutt JG, Fellman JH. Pharmacokinetics of levodopa. Clin Neuropharmacol. 1984;7:35-49.

Robertson DR, Wood ND, Everest H, et al. The effect of age on the pharmacokinetics of levodopa administered alone and in the presence of carbidopa. Br J Clin Pharmacol. 1989;28:61-9.

ANTITHYROID DRUGS

Methimazole

Jansson R, Lindstrom B, Dahlberg PA. Pharmacokinetic properties and bioavailability of methimazole. Clin Pharmacokinet. 1985;10:443-50.

Propylthiouracil

Cooper DS. Antithyroid drugs. N Engl J Med. 1984;311:1353-62.

ARTHRITIS AND GOUT AGENTS

Allopurinol

Hande K, Noone RM, Stone WJ. Severe allopurinol toxicity: description and guidelines for prevention in patients with renal insufficiency. Am J Med. 1984;76:47-56.

Murrell GA, Rappeport WG. Clinical pharmacokinetics of allopurinol. Clin Pharmacokinet. 1986;11:343-53.

Auranofin

Chaffman M, Brogden RN, Heel RC, et al. Auranofin: a preliminary review of its pharmacological properties and therapeutic use in rheumatoid arthritis. Drugs. 1984;27:378-424.

Colchicine

Wallace SL, Omokoku B, Ertel NH. Colchicine plasma levels: implications as to pharmacology and mechanisms of action. Am J Med. 1970;48:443-8.

Wallace SL, Singer JZ, Duncan GJ, et al. Renal function predicts colchicine toxicity. J Rheumatol. 1991;18:264-9.

Gold Sodium Thiomalate

Blocka KL, Paulus HE, Furst DE. Clinical pharmacokinetics of oral and injectable gold compounds. Clin Pharmacokinet. 1986;11:133-43.

Lorber A. Monitoring gold plasma levels in rheumatoid arthritis. Clin Pharmacokinet. 1977;2:127-46.

Penicillamine

Bergstrom RJ, Kay DR, Harkcom TM, et al. Penicillamine kinetics in normal subjects. Clin Pharmacol Ther. 1981;30:404-13.

Lang K. Nephropathy induced by D-penicillamine. Contrib Nephrol. 1978;10:63-74.

Netter P, Bannwarth B, Pere P, et al. Clinical pharmacokinetics of D-penicillamine. Clin Pharmacokinet. 1987;13:317-33.

Probenecid

Cunningham RF, Isaili ZH, Dayton PG. Clinical pharmacokinetics of probenecid. Clin Pharmacokinet. 1981;6:135-51.

Dayton PG, Perel JM. The metabolism of probenecid in man. Ann N Y Acad Sci. 1971;179:399-402.

ARTHRITIS AND GOUT AGENTS: NONSTEROIDAL ANTI-INFLAMMATORY DRUGS

Diclofenac

Todd PA, Sorkin EM. Diclofenac sodium: a reappraisal of its pharmacodynamic and pharmacokinetic properties, and therapeutic efficacy. Drugs. 1988;35:244-85.

Diflunisal

No references

Etodolac

Benet LZ. Pharmacokinetic profile of etodolac in special populations. Eur J Rheumatol Inflamm. 1994;14:15-8.

Fenoprofen

No references

Flurbiprofen

Davies N. Clinical pharmacokinetics of flurbiprofen. Clin Pharmacokinet. 1995;28:100-14.

Ibuprofen

Albert KS, Gernaat CM. Pharmacokinetics of ibuprofen. Am J Med. 1984;77:40-6.

Indomethacin

Helleberg L. Clinical pharmacokinetics of indomethacin. Clin Pharmacokinet. 1981;6:245-58.

Stein G, Kunze M, Zaumseil J, et al. Pharmacokinetics of indomethacin and indomethacin metabolites administered continually to patients with healthy or damaged kidneys. Int J Clin Pharmacol Biopharm. 1977;15:470-3.

Ketoprofen

Skeith KJ, Russell AS, Jamali F. Ketoprofen pharmacokinetics in the elderly. J Clin Pharm. 1993;33:1052-9.

Ketorolac

Buckley M, Brogden RN. Ketorolac. Drugs. 1990;39:86-104.

Otti T, Weindel M, Bastani B. Ketorolac-induced acute reversible hearing loss in a patient maintained on CAPD. Clin Nephrol. 1997;47:208-9.

Meclofenamic Acid

No references

Mefenamic Acid

No references

Nabumetone

No references

Naproxen

Anttila M, Haataja M, Kasanen A. Pharmacokinetics of naproxen in subjects with normal and impaired renal function. Eur J Clin Pharmacol. 1980;18:263-8.

Oxaproxin

No references

Phenylbutazone

Aarbakke J. Clinical pharmacokinetics of phenylbutazone. Clin Pharmacokinet. 1978;3:369-80.

Piroxicam

Brogden RN, Heel RC, Speight TM, et al. Piroxicam: a reappraisal of its pharmacology and therapeutic efficacy. Drugs. 1984;28:292-323.

Olkkola KT, Brunetto AV, Mattila MJ. Pharmacokinetics of oxicam nonsteroidal anti-inflammatory drugs. Clin Pharmacokin. 1994;26:107-20.

Sulindac

Miller MJ, Bednar MM, McGiff JC. Renal metabolism of sulindac: functional implications. J Pharmacol Exp Ther. 1984;231:449-56.

Tolmetin

Selley ML, Glass J, Triggs EG, et al. Pharmacokinetic studies of tolmetin in man. Clin Pharmacol Ther. 1975;17:599-605.

BRONCHODILATORS

Albuterol

Morgan DJ, Paull JD, Richmond BH, et al. Pharmacokinetics of intravenous and oral salbutamol and its sulphate conjugate. Br J Clin Pharmacol. 1986;22:587-93.
Powell ML, Chung M, Weisberger M, et al. Multiple-dose albuterol kinetics. J Clin Pharmacol. 1986;26:643-6.

Dyphylline

Lee CS, Wang LH, Majeske BL, et al. Pharmacokinetics of dyphylline elimination by uremic patients. J Pharmacol Exp Ther. 1981;217:340-4.

Ipratropium

Ensing K, De Zeeuw RA, Nossent GD, et al. Pharmacokinetics of ipratropium bromide after single dose inhalation and oral and intravenous administration. Eur J Clin Pharmacol. 1989;36:189-94.

Metaproterenol

No references

Terbutaline

No references

Theophylline

Hendeles L, Massanari M, Weinberger M. Update on the pharmacodynamics and pharmacokinetics of theophylline. Chest. 1985;88(Suppl 2):103S-11S.
Kradjan WA, Martin TR, Delaney CL, et al. Effect of hemodialysis on the pharmacokinetics of theophylline in chronic renal failure. Nephron. 1982;32:40-4.

BRONCHODILATORS: LEUKOTRIENE INHIBITORS

Zafirlukast

Spector SL, Smith LJ, Glass M, et al. Zafirlukast. Am J Crit Care Med. 1994;150:618-23.

Zileuton

Awni W, Wong S, Chu SY, et al. Pharmacokinetics of zileuton in subjects with renal impairment [Abstract]. Clin Pharmacol Ther. 1997;61:217.

CORTICOSTEROIDS

Betamethasone

No references

Budesonide

No references

Cortisone

No references

Dexamethasone

Brady ME, Sartiano GP, Rosenblum SL, et al. The pharmacokinetics of single high doses of dexamethasone in cancer patients. Eur J Clin Pharmacol. 1987;32:593-6.

Hydrocortisone

No references

Methylprednisolone

Al-Habet SM, Rogers HJ. Methylprednisolone pharmacokinetics after intravenous and oral administration. Br J Clin Pharmacol. 1989;27:285-90.

Prednisolone

Bergrem H. Pharmacokinetics and protein binding of prednisolone in patients with nephrotic syndrome and patients undergoing hemodialysis. Kidney Int. 1983;23:876-81.

Lefler UF, Fre FJ, Benet LZ. Prednisolone clearance at steady state in man. J Clin Endocrinol Metab. 1982;55:762-7.

Pickup ME. Clinical pharmacokinetics of prednisone and prednisolone. Clin Pharmacokinet. 1979;4:111-28.

Prednisone

Bergrem H. Pharmacokinetics and protein binding of prednisolone in patients with nephrotic syndrome and patients undergoing hemodialysis. Kidney Int. 1983;23:876-81.

Lefler UF, Fre FJ, Benet LZ. Prednisolone clearance as steady state in man. J Clin Endocrinol Metab. 1982;55:762-770.

Pickup ME. Clinical pharmacokinetics of prednisone and prednisolone. Clin Pharmacokinet. 1979;4:111-28.

Triamcinolone

Mollmann H, Rohdewald P, Schmidt EW, et al. Pharmacokinetics of triamcinolone acetonide and its phosphate ester. Eur J Clin Pharmacol. 1985;29:85-9.

HYPOGLYCEMIC AGENTS (ORAL)

Acarbose

Balfour JA, McTavish D. Acarbose. Drugs. 1993;46:1025-54.

Acetohexamide

Baba S, Baba T, Iwanaga T. Effect of acetohexamide (a sulfonylurea hypoglycemia agent) in blood plasma on creatinine laboratory tests. Chem Pharm Bull (Tokyo). 1979;27:139-43.

Chlorpropamide

Taylor JA. Pharmacokinetics and biotransformation of chlorpropamide in man. Clin Pharmacol Ther. 1972;13:710-8.

Glibornuride

No references

Gliclazide

Holmes B, Heel RC, Brogden RN, et al. Gliclazide: a preliminary review of its pharmacodynamic properties and therapeutic efficacy in diabetes mellitus. Drugs. 1984;27:301-27.
Palmer KJ, Brogden RN. Glicazide. Drugs. 1993;46:92-125.

Glipizide

Lebovitz HE. Glipizide: a second generation sulfonylurea hypoglycemic agent: pharmacology, pharmacokinetics and clinical use. Pharmacotherapy. 1985;5:63-77.
Wensing G. Topics in clinical pharmacology. Glipizide: an oral hypoglycemic drug. Am J Med Sci. 1989;298:69-71.

Glyburide

Feldman JM. Glyburide: a second generation sulfonylurea hypoglycemic agent. History, chemistry, metabolism, pharmacokinetics, clinical use and adverse effects. Pharmacotherapy. 1985;5:43-62.

Metformin

Dunn CJ, Peters DH. Metformin. Drugs. 1995;49:121-49.

Tolazamide

No references

Tolbutamide

Nelson E. Rate of metabolism of tolbutamide in test subjects with liver disease or with impaired renal function. Am J Med Sci. 1964;248:657-9.

HYPOGLYCEMIC AGENTS (PARENTERAL)

Insulin

Brogden RN, Heel RC. Human insulin: a review of its biological activity, pharmacokinetics and therapeutic use. Drugs. 1987;34:350-71.

Rabkin R, Simon NM, Steinder S, et al. Effect of renal disease on renal uptake and excretion of insulin in man. N Engl J Med. 1970;282:182-7.

Lispro Insulin

Howey DC, Browsher R, Brunelle R, et al. LysPro human insulin. Diabetes. 1994;43:396-99.

HYPOLIPIDEMIC AGENTS

Bezafibrate

Goa KL, Barradell LB, Plosker GL. Bezafibrate. Drugs. 1996;52:725-53.

Monk JP, Todd PA. Bezafibrate: a review of its pharmacodynamic and pharmacokinetic properties, and therapeutic use in hyperlipidaemia. Drugs. 1987;33:539-76.

Cholestyramine

Silverberg DS, Iaina A, Reisin E, et al. Cholestyramine in uremic pruritis. BMJ. 1977;1:752-3.

Clofibrate

Gugler R. Clinical pharmacokinetics of hypolipidaemic drugs. Clin Pharmacokinet. 1978;3:425-39.

Colestipol

No references

Fluvastatin

Jokubaitis LA. Updated clinical safety experience with fluvastatin. Am J Cardiol. 1994;73:18D-24D.

Gemfibrozil

Manninen V, Malkonen M, Eisalo A. Gemfibrozil treatment of dyslipidaemias in renal failure with uremia or in the nephrotic syndrome. Res Clin Forums. 1982;4:113-8.

Todd PA, Ward A. Gemfibrozil: a review of its pharmacodynamic and pharmacokinetic properties, and therapeutic use in dyslipidaemia. Drugs. 1988;36:314-39.

Lovastatin

Henwood JM, Heel RC. Lovastatin: a preliminary review of its pharmacodynamic properties and therapeutic use in hyperlipidaemia. Drugs. 1988;36:429-54.

Nicotinic Acid

Gokal R, Mann JI, Oliver DO, et al. Treatment of hyperlipidemia in patients on chronic hemodialysis. BMJ. 1978;1:82-3.

Pravastatin

Halstenson CE, Triscari J, DeVault A, et al. Single dose pharmacokinetics of pravastatin in patients with renal insufficiency. J Clin Pharm. 1992;32:124-32.

Probucol

No references

Simvastatin

Plosker GL, McTavish D. Simvastatin. Drugs. 1995;50:334-63.

MISCELLANEOUS DRUGS (VARIOUS)

Acetohydroxamic Acid

Lake KD, Brown DC. New drug therapy for kidney stones: a review of cellulose sodium phosphate, acetohydroxamic acid, and potassium citrate. Drug Intell Clin Pharm. 1985;19:530-9.

N-Acetylcysteine

Borgstrom L, Kagedal B, Paulsen O. Pharmacokinetics of *N*-acetylcysteine in man. Eur J Clin Pharmacol. 1986;31:217-22.

Cisapride

Wiseman LR, Faulds D. Cisapride. Drugs. 1994;47:116-52.

Clodronate

Conrad KA, Lee SM. Clondronate kinetics and dynamics. Clin Pharmacol Ther. 1981;30:114-20.
Saha H, Castrem-Kortekangas P, Ojanen S, et al. Pharmacokinetics of clodronate in renal failure. J Bone Mineral Res. 1994;9:1953-8.

Cyclosporine

Awni WM, Kasiske BL, Heim-Duthoy K, et al. Long-term cyclosporine pharmacokinetic changes in renal transplant recipients: effects of binding and metabolism. Clin Pharmacol Ther. 1989;45:41-8.

Fullath F, Wenk M, Vozeh S, et al. Intravenous cyclosporine kinetics in renal failure. Clin Pharmacol Ther. 1983;34:638-43.

Rodighiero V. Therapeutic drug monitoring of cyclosporine: practical applications and limitations. Clin Pharmacokinet. 1989;16:27-37.

Desferoxamine

Allain P, Morass Y, Chill D, et al. Pharmacokinetics and renal elimination of desferrioxamine and ferrioxamine in healthy subjects and patients with haemochromatosis. Br J Clin Pharmacol. 1987;24:207-12.

Metoclopramide

Bateman DN. Clinical pharmacokinetics of metoclopramide. Clin Pharmacokinet. 1983;8:523-9.

Ondansetron

Wilde M, Markham A. Ondansetron. Drugs. 1996;52:773-94.

Pentoxifylline

Baker DE, Campbell RK. Pentoxifylline: a new agent for intermittent claudication. Drug Intell Clin Pharm. 1985;19:345-8.

Beermann B, Ings R, Mansby J, et al. Kinetics of intravenous and oral pentoxifylline in healthy subjects. Clin Pharmacol Ther. 1985;37:25-8.

Paap CM, Simpson KS, Horton MW, et al. Multiple dose pharmacokinetics of pentoxifylline and its metabolites in renal insufficiency. Ann Pharmacother. 1996;30:724-9.

Ward A, Clissold SP. Pentoxifylline: a review of its pharmacodynamic and pharmacokinetic properties, and its therapeutic efficacy. Drugs. 1987;34:50-97.

NEUROMUSCULAR AGENTS

Alcuronium

Difenbach C, Thomas K, Buzello CW, et al. Alcuronium pharmacodynamic and pharmacokinetic update. Anesth Analg. 1995;80:373-7.

Alfentanil

Van Peer A, Vercauteren M, Noorduin H, et al. Alfentanil kinetics in renal insufficiency. Eur J Clin Pharmacol. 1986;30:245-7.

Atracurium

Conner CS. Atracurium and vecuronium: two unique neuromuscular blocking agents. Drug Intell Clin Pharm. 1984;18:714-6.

Shearer ES, O'Sullivan EP, Hunter JM. Clearance of atracurium and laudanosine in the urine and by continuous venovenous haemofiltration. Br J Anaesth. 1991;67:569-73.

Doxacurium

Cook DR, Freeman JA, Lai AA, et al. Pharmacokinetics and pharmacodynamics of doxacurium in normal patients and in those with hepatic or renal failure. Anesth Analg. 1991;72:145-50.

Etomidate

No references

Fazadinium

Bevan DR, D'Souza J, Rouse KM, et al. Clinical pharmacokinetics and pharmacodynamics of fazadinium in renal failure. Eur J Clin Pharmacol. 1981;20:293-8.

Smith CE, Hunter JM. Anesthesia for renal transplantation-relaxants and volatiles. Int Anesth Clin. 1996;33:69-92.

Fentanyl

Mather LE. Clinical pharmacokinetics of fentanyl and its newer derivatives. Clin Pharmacokinet. 1983;8:422-46.

Gallamine

Ramzan MI, Shanks CA, Triggs EJ. Gallamine disposition in surgical patients with chronic renal failure. J Clin Pharmacol. 1981;12:141-7.

Ketamine

No references

Metocurine

No references

Mivacurium

Phillips BJ, Hunter JM. Use of mivacurium chloride by constant infusion in the anephric patient. Br J Anaesth. 1992;68:492-8.

Neostigmine

Cronnelly R, Stanski DR, Miller RD, et al. Renal function and the pharmacokinetics of neostigmine in anesthetized man. Anesthesiology. 1979;51:222-6.

Pancuronium

McLeod K, Watson MJ, Rawlings MD. Pharmacokinetics of pancuronium in patients with normal and impaired renal function. Br J Anaesth. 1976;48:341-5.

Pipecuronium

Caldwell JE, Canfell PC, Castagnoli KP, et al. The influence of renal failure on the pharmacokinetics and duration of action of pipercuronium bromide in patients anesthetized with halothane and nitrous oxide. Anesthesiology. 1989;70:7-12.

Propofol

Nathan N, Debord J, Narcisse F, et al. Pharmacokinetics of propofol and its conjugates after continuous infusion in normal and in renal failure patients. Acta Anaesthesiol Belg. 1993;44:77-85.

Pyridostigmine

Cronnelly R, Stanski DR, Miller RD, et al. Pyridostigmine kinetics with and without renal function. Clin Pharmacol Ther. 1980;28:78-81.

Succinylcholine

Bishop M, Hornbein TF. Prolonged effect of succinylcholine after neostigmine and pyridostigmine administration in patients with renal failure. Anesthesiology. 1983;58:384-6.

Sufentanil

Monk JP, Beresford R, Ward A. Sufentanil: a review of its pharmacological properties and therapeutic use. Drugs. 1988;36:286-313.

Tubocurarine

Miller RD, Matteo RS, Benet LZ, et al. The pharmacokinetics of D-tubocurarine in man with and without renal failure. J Pharmacol Exp Ther. 1977;202:1-7.

Vecuronium

Miller RD. Vecuronium: a new nondepolarizing neuromuscular-blocking agent: clinical pharmacology, pharmacokinetics, cardiovascular effects and use in special clinical situations. Pharmacotherapy. 1984;4:238-47.

Shanks CA, Avram MJ, Fragen RJ, et al. Pharmacokinetics and pharmacodynamics of vecuronium administered by bolus and infusion during holothane or balanced anesthesia. Clin Pharmacol Ther. 1987;42:459-64.

PROTON-PUMP INHIBITORS

Lansoprazole

Karol MD, Machinist JM, Cavanaugh JM. Lansoprazole pharmacokinetics in subjects with various degrees of kidney function. Clin Pharmacol Ther. 1997;61:450-8.

Spencer CM, Faulds D. Lansoprazole. Drugs. 1994;48:404-30.

Omeprazole

Naesdal J, Anderson T, Bodemar G, et al. Pharmacokinetics of [14C] omeprazole in patients with impaired renal function. Clin Pharmacol Ther. 1986;40:344-51.

Sedatives, Hypnotics, and Other Drugs Used in Psychiatry

ANTIDEPRESSANTS

Bupropion

DeVane CL. Pharmacokinetics of the selective serotonin reuptake inhibitors [Review]. J Clin Psychiatry. 1992;53(Suppl):13-20.

DeVane CL. Pharmacokinetics of the newer antidepressants: clinical relevance. Am J Med. 1994;97(Suppl 6A):13S-23S.

Goodnick PJ. Pharmacokinetics of second generation antidepressants: bupropion. Psychopharmacol Bull. 1991;27:513-9.

Laizure SC, Devane CL, Stewart JJ, et al. Pharmacokinetics of bupropion and its major basic metabolite in normal subjects after single dose. Clin Pharmacol Ther. 1985;38:586-9.

Posner J, Bye A, Dean K, et al. Disposition of bupropion and its metabolism in healthy male volunteers after single dose and multiple doses. Eur J Clin Pharmacol. 1985;29:97-103.

Nefazodone

DeVane CL. Pharmacokinetics of the newer antidepressants: clinical relevance. Am J Med. 1994;97(Suppl 6A):13S-23S.

Ellingrod VL, Perry PJ. Nefazodone: a new antidepressant. Am J Health Syst Pharm. 1995;52:2799-812.

Goldberg RJ. Nefazodone and venlaflaxine: two new agents for the treatment of depression. J Fam Pract. 1995;41:5914.

Preskorn SH. Comparison of the tolerability of bupropion, fluoxetine, imipramine, nefazodone, paroxetine, sertraline, and venlafaxine. J Clin Psychiatry. 1995;56(Suppl 6):12-21.

Trazodone

Browne TR. The pharmacokinetics of agents used to treat status epilepticus [Review]. Neurology. 1990;40(Suppl 2):28-32.

DeVane CL. Pharmacokinetics of the newer antidepressants: clinical relevance. Am J Med. 1994;97(Suppl 6A):13S-23S.

Preskorn SH. Comparison of the tolerability of bupropion, fluoxetine, imipramine, nefazodone, paroxetine, sertraline, and venlafaxine. J Clin Psychiatry. 1995;56(Suppl 6):12-21.

Venlafaxine

DeVane CL. Pharmacokinetics of the newer antidepressants: clinical relevance. Am J Med. 1994;97(Suppl 6A):13S-23S.

Ellingrod VL, Perry PJ. Venlaflaxine: a heterocyclic antidepressant. Am J Hosp Pharm. 1994;51:3033-46.

Holliday SM, Benfield P. Venlafaxine: a review of its pharmacology and therapeutic potential in depression. Drugs. 1995;49:280-94.

Morton WA, Sonne SC, Verga MA. Venlafaxine: a structurally unique and novel antidepressant. Ann Pharmacother. 1995;29:387-95.

Preskorn SH. Comparison of the tolerability of bupropion, fluoxetine, imipramine, nefazodone, paroxetine, sertraline, and venlafaxine. J Clin Psychiatry. 1995;56(Suppl 6):12-21.

Scott MA, Shelton PS, Gattis W. Therapeutic options for treating major depression and the role of venlaflaxine. Pharmacotherapy. 1996;16:352-65.

BARBITURATES

Pentobarbital

Browne TR. The pharmacokinetics of agents used to treat status epilepticus [Review]. Neurology. 1990;40(Suppl 2):28-32.

Wermeling D, Record K, Bell R, et al. Hemodialysis clearance of pentobarbital during continuous infusion. Ther Drug Monit. 1985;7:485-7.

Phenobarbital

Browne TR. The pharmacokinetics of agents used to treat status epilepticus [Review]. Neurology. 1990;40(Suppl 2):28-32.

Mattson RH. Parenteral antiepileptic/anticonvulsant drugs. Neurology. 1996;46(Suppl 1):S8-13.

Riva R, Albani F, Contin M, et al. Pharmacokinetic interactions between antiepileptic drugs: clinical considerations. Clin Pharmacokinet. 1996;31:470-93.

Rogvi-Hansen B, Gram L. Adverse effects of established and antiepileptic drugs: an attempted comparison. Pharmacol Ther. 1995;68:425-34.

Shihab-Eldeen AA, Peck GE, Ash SR, Kaufman G. Evaluation of the sorbent suspension reciprocating dialyser in the treatment of overdose of paracetamol and phenobarbitone. J Pharm Pharmacol. 1988;40:381-7.

Secobarbital

Browne TR. The pharmacokinetics of agents used to treat status epilepticus [Review]. Neurology. 1990;40(Suppl 2):28-32.

Thiopental

Browne TR. The pharmacokinetics of agents used to treat status epilepticus [Review]. Neurology. 1990;40(Suppl 2):28-32.

BENZODIAZEPINES

Laurijssens BE, Greenblatt DJ. Pharmacokinetic-pharmacodynamic relationships for benzodiazepines. Clin Pharmacokinet. 1996;30:52-76.

Murray MJ, DeRuyter ML, Harrison BA. Opioids and benzodiazepines. Crit Care Clin. 1995;11:849-73.

Vgontzas AN, Kales A, Bixler EO. Benzodiazepine side effects: role of pharmacokinetics and pharmacodynamics. Pharmacology (Berl). 1995;51:205-23.

Woods JH, Winger G. Current benzodiazepine issues. Psychopharmacology (Berl). 1995;118:107-15.

Alprazolam

Devane CL, Ware MR, Lydlard RB. Pharmacokinetics, pharmacodynamics and treatment issues for benzodiazepines: alprazolam, adinazolam and clonazepam. Psychopharmacol Bull. 1991;27:463-73.

Greenblatt DJ. Benzodiazepine hypnotics: sorting the pharmacokinetic facts [Review]. J Clin Psychiatry. 1991;52(Suppl):4-10.

Greenblatt DJ. Pharmacokinetics and pharmacodynamics [Review]. Hosp Pract. 1990;25(Suppl 2):9-15.

Greenblatt DJ, Harmatz JS, Dorsey C, et al. Comparative single dose kinetics and dynamics of lorazepam, alprazolam, prazepam, and placebo. Clin Pharmacol Ther. 1988;44:326-34.

Chlordiazepoxide

Gaudreault P, Guay J, Thivierge RL, et al. Benzodiazepine poisoning: clinical and pharmacological considerations and treatment [Review]. Drug Safety. 1991;6:247-65.

Greenblatt DJ. Pharmacokinetics and pharmacodynamics [Review]. Hosp Pract. 1990;25(Suppl 2):9-15.

Greenblatt DJ. Benzodiazepine hypnotics: sorting the pharmacokinetic facts [Review]. J Clin Psychiatry. 1991;52(Suppl):4-10.

Clonazepam

Gaudreault P, Guay J, Thivierge RL, et al. Benzodiazepine poisoning: clinical and pharmacological considerations and treatment [Review]. Drug Safety. 1991;6:247-65.

Greenblatt DJ. Pharmacokinetics and pharmacodynamics [Review]. Hosp Pract. 1990;25(Suppl 2):9-15.

Greenblatt DJ. Benzodiazepine hypnotics: sorting the pharmacokinetic facts [Review]. J Clin Psychiatry. 1991;52(Suppl):4-10.

Trelman DM. Pharmacokinetics and clinical use of benzodiazepines in the management of status epilepticus [Review]. Epilepsia. 1989;30(Suppl 2):S4-10.

Clorazepate

Duguay R. Efficacy and kinetics of clorazepate administered to anxious patients in a single daily dose. Can J Psychiatry. 1985;30:414-7.

Gaudreault P, Guay J, Thivierge RL, et al. Benzodiazepine poisoning: clinical and pharmacological considerations and treatment [Review]. Drug Safety. 1991;6:247-65.

Greenblatt DJ. Benzodiazepine hypnotics: sorting the pharmacokinetic facts [Review]. J Clin Psychiatry. 1991;52(Suppl):4-10.

Greenblatt DJ. Pharmacokinetics and pharmacodynamics [Review]. Hosp Pract. 1990;25(Suppl 2):9-15.

Diazepam

Gaudreault P, Guay J, Thivierge RL, et al. Benzodiazepine poisoning: clinical and pharmacological considerations and treatment [Review]. Drug Safety. 1991;6:247-65.

Greenblatt DJ. Pharmacokinetics and pharmacodynamics [Review]. Hosp Pract. 1990;25(Suppl 2):9-15.

Greenblatt DJ. Benzodiazepine hypnotics: sorting the pharmacokinetic facts [Review]. J Clin Psychiatry. 1991;52(Suppl):4-10.
Greenblatt DJ, Harmatz JS, Friedman H, et al. A large sample study of diazepam pharmacokinetics. Ther Drug Monit. 1989;11:652-7.
Trelman DM. Pharmacokinetics and clinical use of benzodiazepines in the management of status epilepticus [Review]. Epilepsia. 1989;30(Suppl 2):S4-10.
Vanholder R, Van-Landschoot N, DeSmet R, et al. Drug protein binding in chronic renal failure: evaluation of nine drugs. Kidney Int. 1990;33:996-1004.

Estazolam

Gaudreault P, Guay J, Thivierge RL, et al. Benzodiazepine poisoning: clinical and pharmacological considerations and treatment [Review]. Drug Safety. 1991;6:247-65.
Greenblatt DJ. Pharmacokinetics and pharmacodynamics [Review]. Hosp Pract. 1990;25(Suppl 2):9-15.
Greenblatt DJ. Benzodiazepine hypnotics: sorting the pharmacokinetic facts [Review]. J Clin Psychiat. 1991;52(Suppl):4-10.
Gustavson LE, Carrigan PJ. The clinical pharmacokinetics of a single dose of estazolam. Am J Med. 1990;88(3A):2S-5S.
Trelman DM. Pharmacokinetics and clinical use of benzodiazepines in the management of status epilepticus [Review]. Epilepsia. 1989;30(Suppl 2):S4-10.

Flurazepam

Gaudreault P, Guay J, Thivierge RL, et al. Benzodiazepine poisoning: clinical and pharmacological considerations and treatment [Review]. Drug Safety. 1991;6:247-65.
Greenblatt DJ. Pharmacokinetics and pharmacodynamics [Review]. Hosp Pract. 1990;25(Suppl 2):9-15.
Greenblatt DJ. Benzodiazepine hypnotics: sorting the pharmacokinetic facts [Review]. J Clin Psychiatry. 1991;52(Suppl):4-10.
Greenblatt DJ, Harmatz JS, Engelhardt N, et al. Pharmacokinetic determinants of dynamic differences among three benzodiazepine hypnotics: flurazepam, temazepam, and triazolam. Arch Gen Psychiat. 1989;46:326-32.
Trelman DM. Pharmacokinetics and clinical use of benzodiazepines in the management of status epilepticus [Review]. Epilepsia. 1989;30(Suppl 2):S4-10.

Lorazepam

Gaudreault P, Guay J, Thivierge RL, et al. Benzodiazepine poisoning: clinical and pharmacological considerations and treatment [Review]. Drug Safety. 1991;6:247-65.
Greenblatt DJ. Pharmacokinetics and pharmacodynamics [Review]. Hosp Pract. 1990;25(Suppl 2):9-15.
Greenblatt DJ. Benzodiazepine hypnotics: sorting the pharmacokinetic facts [Review]. J Clin Psychiat. 1991;52(Suppl):4-10.
Greenblatt DJ, Ehrenberg BL, Gunderman J, et al. Kinetic and dynamic study of intravenous lorazepam: comparison with intravenous diazepam. J Pharmacol Exp Ther. 1989;250:134-40.
Greenblatt DJ, Harmatz JS, Dorsey C, et al. Comparative single-dose kinetics and dynamics of lorazepam, alprazolam, prazepam, and placebo. Clin Pharmacol Ther. 1988;44:326-34.
Trelman DM. Pharmacokinetics and clinical use of benzodiazepines in the management of status epilepticus [Review]. Epilepsia. 1989;30(Suppl 2):S4-10.

Midazolam

Bell DM, Richards G, Phillon S, et al. A comparative pharmacokinetic study of intravenous and intramuscular midazolam in patients with epilepsy. Epilepsy Res. 1991;10:183-90.

Castelden CM, Allen JG, Altman J, et al. A comparison of oral midazolam, nitrazepam and placebo in young and elderly subjects. Eur J Clin Pharmacol. 1987;32:253-7.

Crevat-Pisano P, Dragna S, Granthil C, et al. Plasma concentrations and pharmacokinetics of midazolam during anaesthesia. J Pharma Pharmacol. 1986;38:578-82.

Gaudreault P, Guay J, Thivierge RL, et al. Benzodiazepine poisoning: clinical and pharmacological considerations and treatment [Review]. Drug Safety. 1991;6:247-65.

Greenblatt DJ. Pharmacokinetics and pharmacodynamics [Review]. Hosp Pract. 1990;25(Suppl 2):9-15.

Greenblatt DJ. Benzodiazepine hypnotics: sorting the pharmacokinetic facts [Review]. J Clin Psychiat. 1991;52(Suppl):4-10.

Trelman DM. Pharmacokinetics and clinical use of benzodiazepines in the management of status epilepticus [Review]. Epilepsia. 1989;30(Suppl 2):S4-10.

Oxazepam

Ayd FJ Jr. Oxazepam: update 1989. Int Clin Psychopharmacol. 1990;5:1-15.

Gaudreault P, Guay J, Thivierge RL, et al. Benzodiazepine poisoning: clinical and pharmacological considerations and treatment [Review]. Drug Safety. 1991;6:247-65.

Greenblatt DJ. Pharmacokinetics and pharmacodynamics [Review]. Hosp Pract. 1990;25(Suppl 2):9-15.

Greenblatt DJ. Benzodiazepine hypnotics: sorting the pharmacokinetic facts [Review]. J Clin Psychiat. 1991;52(Suppl):4-10.

Sonne J, Loft S, Dossing M, et al. Bioavailability and pharmacokinetics of oxazepam. Eur J Clin Pharmacol. 1988;35:385-9.

Trelman DM. Pharmacokinetics and clinical use of benzodiazepines in the management of status epilepticus [Review]. Epilepsia. 1989;30(Suppl 2):S4-10.

Quazepam

Gaudreault P, Guay J, Thivierge RL, et al. Benzodiazepine poisoning: clinical and pharmacological considerations and treatment [Review]. Drug Safety. 1991;6:247-65.

Greenblatt DJ. Pharmacokinetics and pharmacodynamics [Review]. Hosp Pract. 1990;25(Suppl 2):9-15.

Greenblatt DJ. Benzodiazepine hypnotics: sorting the pharmacokinetic facts [Review]. J Clin Psychiat. 1991;52(Suppl):4-10.

Hilbert JM, Battista D. Quazepam and flurazepam: differential pharmacokinetics and pharmacodynamic characteristics. J Clin Psychiatry. 1991;52:21-6.

Temazepam

Gaudreault P, Guay J, Thivierge RL, et al. Benzodiazepine poisoning: clinical and pharmacological considerations and treatment [Review]. Drug Safety. 1991;6:247-65.

Greenblatt DJ. Pharmacokinetics and pharmacodynamics [Review]. Hosp Pract. 1990;25(Suppl 2):9-15.

Greenblatt DJ. Benzodiazepine hypnotics: sorting the pharmacokinetic facts [Review]. J Clin Psychiat. 1991;52(Suppl):4-10.

Greenblatt DJ, Harmatz JS, Engelhardt N, et al. Pharmacokinetic determinants of dynamic differences among three benzodiazepine hypnotics: flurazepam, temazepam, and triazolam. Arch Gen Psychiat. 1989;46:326-32.

Krobath PD, Smith RB, Rault R, et al. Effects of end-stage renal disease and aluminum hydroxide on temazepam kinetics. Clin Pharmacol Ther. 1985;37:453-9.

Triazolam

Friedman H, Greenblatt DJ, Burstein ES, et al. Population study of triazolam pharmacokinetics. Br J Clin Pharmacol. 1986;22:639-42.

Gaudreault P, Guay J, Thivierge RL, et al. Benzodiazepine poisoning: clinical and pharmacological considerations and treatment [Review]. Drug Safety. 1991;6:247-65.

Greenblatt DJ. Pharmacokinetics and pharmacodynamics [Review]. Hosp Pract. 1990;25(Suppl 2):9-15.

Greenblatt DJ. Benzodiazepine hypnotics: sorting the pharmacokinetic facts [Review]. J Clin Psychiat. 1991;52(Suppl):4-10.

Greenblatt DJ, Harmatz JS, Engelhardt N, et al. Pharmacokinetic determinants of dynamic differences among three benzodiazepine hypnotics: flurazepam, temazepam, and triazolam. Arch Gen Psychiat. 1989;46:326-32.

Kroboth PD, Smith RB, Silver MR, et al. Effects of end-stage renal disease and aluminum hydroxide on triazolam pharmacokinetics. Br J Clin Pharmacol. 1985;19:839-42.

Trelman DM. Pharmacokinetics and clinical use of benzodiazepines in the management of status epilepticus [Review]. Epilepsia. 1989;30(Suppl 2):S4-10.

BENZODIAZEPINES: BENZODIAZEPINE ANTAGONIST

Flumazenil

Brogden RN, Goa KL. Flumazenil: a reappraisal of its pharmacological properties and therapeutic efficacy as a benzodiazepine antagonist. Drugs. 1991;42:1061-89.

Gaudreault P, Guay J, Thivierge RL, et al. Benzodiazepine poisoning: clinical and pharmacological considerations and treatment [Review]. Drug Safety. 1991;6:247-65.

Greenblatt DJ. Pharmacokinetics and pharmacodynamics [Review]. Hosp Pract. 1990;25(Suppl 2):9-15.

Greenblatt DJ. Benzodiazepine hypnotics: sorting the pharmacokinetic facts [Review]. J Clin Psychiat. 1991;52(Suppl):4-10.

Karavokiros KA, Tsipis GB. Flumazenil: a benzodiazepine antagonist. DICP. 1990;24:976-81.

Trelman DM. Pharmacokinetics and clinical use of benzodiazepines in the management of status epilepticus [Review]. Epilepsia. 1989;30(Suppl 2):S4-10.

Vetey SR, Bosse GM, Boyer MJ, et al. Flumazenil: a new benzodiazepine antagonist. Ann Emerg Med. 1991;20:181-8.

MISCELLANEOUS SEDATIVE AGENTS

Buspirone

Caccia S, Vigano GL, Mingardi G, et al. Clinical pharmacokinetics of oral buspirone in patients with impaired renal function. Clin Pharmacokinet. 1988;14:171-7.

Dommisse CE, Devane CL. Buspirone: a new type of anxiolytic [Review]. Drug Intell Clin Pharm. 1985;19:624-8.

Eison AS, Temple DL. Buspirone: review of its pharmacology and current perspectives on its mechanisms of action. Am J Med. 1986;80:1-9.

Gammans RE, Mayol RJ, Labudde JA. Metabolism and disposition of buspirone. Am J Med. 1986;80:41-51.

Goa KL, Ward A. Buspirone: a preliminary review of its pharmacological properties and therapeutic efficacy as an anxiolytic [Review]. Drugs. 1986;32:114-29.

Gulyassy PF, Depner TA. Impaired binding of drugs and endogenous ligands in renal diseases. Am J Kid Dis. 1983;2:578-601.

Pecknold JC. A risk-benefit assessment of buspirone in the treatment of anxiety disorders. Drug Safety. 1997;16:118-32.

Ethchlorvynol

Yell RP. Ethchlorvynol overdose. Am J Emerg Med. 1990;8:246-50.

Haloperidol

Fruemming JS, Lam YH, Jann MW, et al. Pharmacokinetics of haloperidol. Clin Pharmacokinet. 1989;17:396-423.

Lithium Carbonate

Arancibia A, Corvalan F, Mella F, et al. Absorption and disposition kinetics of lithium carbonate following administration of conventional and controlled release formulations. Int J Clin Pharmacol Ther Toxicol. 1986;24:240-5.

Hardy BG, Shulman KI, Mackenzie SE, et al. Pharmacokinetics of lithium in the elderly. J Clin Psychopharmacol. 1987;7:153-8.

Luisier PA, Schultz P, Dick P. The pharmacokinetics of lithium in normal humans: expected and unexpected observations in view of basic kinetic principles. Pharmacopsychiatry. 1987;20:232-4.

Shelley RK, Silverstone T. Single dose pharmacokinetics of 5 formulations of lithium: a controlled comparison in healthy subjects. Int Clin Psychopharmacol. 1986;1:324-31.

Thornhill DP. Serum levels and pharmacokinetics of ordinary and sustained-release lithium carbonate in manic patients during chronic dosage. Int J Clin Pharmacol Ther Toxicol. 1986;24:257-61.

Meprobamate

Hassan E. Treatment of meprobamate overdose with repeated oral doses of activated charcoal. Ann Emerg Med. 1986;15:73-6.

Jacobsen D, Wiik-Larsen E, Saltvedt E, et al. Meprobamate kinetics during and after terminated hemoperfusion in acute intoxications. J Toxicol Clin Toxicol. 1987;25:317-31.

PHENOTHIAZINES

Chlorpromazine

Indraprarsit S, Sooksriwongse C. Effect of chlorpromazine on peritoneal clearances. Nephron. 1985;40:341-3.

Verbeeck RK, Cardinal JA. Plasma protein binding of salicylic acid, phenytoin, chlorpromazine, propranalol, and pethidine using equilibrium dialysis and ultracentrifugation. Arzneimittelforschung. 1985;35:903-6.

Promethazine

Stavchansky S, Wallace JE, Geary R, et al. Bioequivalance and pharmacokinetic profile of promethazine hydrochloride suppositories in humans. J Pharm Sci. 1987;76:441-5.

SELECTIVE SEROTONIN-REUPTAKE INHIBITORS (SSRIS)

Fluoxetine

Altamuira AC, Moro AR, Percudani M. Clinical pharmacokinetics of fluoxetine. Clin Pharmacokinet. 1994;26:201-14.

Gam LF. Fluoxetine. N Eng J Med. 1994;331:1354-61.

Goodnick PJ. Pharmacokinetic optimisation of therapy with newer antidepressants. Clin Pharmacokinet. 1994;27:307-30.

Sussman N, Stahl S. Update in the pharmacotherapy of depression. Am J Med. 1996;101(Suppl 6A):26S-36S.

Fluvoxamine

Harten JV. Overview of the pharmacokinetics of fluvoxamine. Clin Pharmacokinet. 1995;29(Suppl 1):1-9.

Perucca E, Gatti G, Spina E. Clinical pharmacokinetics of fluvoxamine. Clin Pharmacokinet. 1994;27:175-90.

Paroxetine

Nemeroff CB. The clinical pharmacology and use of paroxetine, a new selective serotonin re-uptake inhibitor. Pharmacotherapy. 1994;14(2):127-38.

Sertraline

Cohen LJ. Rational drug use in the treatment of depression. Pharmacotherapy. 1997;17:45-61.

TRICYCLIC ANTIDEPRESSANTS

Amitriptyline

Sallee FR, Pollock BG. Clinical pharmacokinetics of imipramine and desipramine. Clin Pharmacokinet. 1990;18:346-64.

Tassett JJ, Singh S, Pesce AJ. Evaluation of amitriptyline pharmacokinetics during peritoneal dialysis. Ther Drug Monit. 1985;7:255-7.

Amoxapine

Calvo B, Garcia MJ, Pedraz JL, et al. Pharmacokinetics of amoxapine and its active metabolites and apparent drug resistance. Int J Clin Pharmacol Ther Toxicol. 1985;23:180-5.

Clomipramine

Sallee FR, Pollock BG. Clinical pharmacokinetics of imipramine and desipramine. Clin Pharmacokinet. 1990;18:346-64.

Desipramine

Kennedy SH, Craven JL, Roin GM. Major depression in renal dialysis patients: an open trial of antidepressant therapy. J Clin Psychiat. 1989;50:60-3.
Sallee FR, Pollock BG. Clinical pharmacokinetics of imipramine and desipramine. Clin Pharmacokinet. 1990;18:346-64.

Doxepin

Coccaro EF, Siever LJ. Second generation antidepressants: a comparative review [Review]. J Clin Pharmacol. 1985;25:241-60.
El-Yazigi A, Chaleby K. Steady-state kinetics of doxepin and imipramine in Saudi patients with interethnic comparison [Review]. Psychopharmacology (Berl). 1988;95:63-7.
Sallee FR, Pollock BG. Clinical pharmacokinetics of imipramine and desipramine. Clin Pharmacokinet. 1990;18:346-64.

Imipramine

Bickel MH, Raaflaub RM, Hellmuller M, et al. Characterization of drug distribution and binding competition by two-chamber and multichamber distribution dialysis. J Pharm Sci. 1987;76:68-74.
El-Yazigi A, Chaleby K. Steady-state kinetics of doxepin and imipramine in Saudi patients with interethnic comparison [Review]. Psychopharmacology (Berl). 1988;95:63-7.
Lieberman JA, Cooper TB, Suckow RF, et al. Tricyclic antidepressant and metabolite levels in chronic renal failure. Clin Pharmacol Ther. 1985;37:301-7.
Sallee FR, Pollock BG. Clinical pharmacokinetics of imipramine and desipramine. Clin Pharmacokinet. 1990;18:346-64.

Nortriptyline

El-Yazigi A, Chaleby K. Steady-state concentrations of amitriptyline and its metabolite nortriptyline in Saudi patients. Ther Drug Monit. 1987;9:6-10.
Sallee FR, Pollock BG. Clinical pharmacokinetics of imipramine and desipramine. Clin Pharmacokinet. 1990;18:346-64.

Protryptyline

Sallee FR, Pollock BG. Clinical pharmacokinetics of imipramine and desipramine. Clin Pharmacokinet. 1990;18:346-64.

Trimipramine

Von Moltke LL, Greenblatt DJ, Shader RI. Clinical pharmacokinetics of antidepressants in the elderly: therapeutic implications. Clin Pharmacokinet. 1993;24:141-60.

Index to Tables and Bibliography

Colchicine, 77, 150
Colestipol, 85
Corticosteroids, 81-83, 153-154
Cortisone, 82
Cyclophosphamide, 73, 145
Cycloserine, 56
Cyclosporine, 87, 156-157
Cytarabine, 73, 145

Dapsone, 48, 123
Daunorubicin, 73, 145
Delavirdine, 59
Desferoxamine, 87, 157
Desipramine, 97, 168
Dexamethasone, 82, 153
Diazepam, 93, 162-163
Diazoxide, 30, 107
Diclofenac, 78, 150
Dicloxacillin, 51, 128
Didanosine, 59, 136
Diflunisal, 78
Digitoxin, 34, 112
Digoxin, 34, 112
Dilevalol, 28, 106
Diltiazem, 33, 110
Diphenhydramine, 69
Dipyridamole, 65, 139
Dirithromycin, 48, 123
Disopyramide, 31, 109
Diuretics, 35-36, 112-114
Dobutamine, 37, 114
Doxacurium, 87, 158
Doxazosin, 24, 102
Doxepin, 97, 168
Doxorubicin, 73, 146
Doxycycline, 54
Dyphylline, 80, 152

Enalapril, 26, 104
Epirubicin, 73, 146
Erbastine, 69, 143
Erythromycin, 48, 123
Esmolol, 29, 106
Estazolam, 93, 163
Ethacrynic acid, 35, 113
Ethambutol, 56, 134
Ethchlorvynol, 95, 166
Ethionamide, 56
Ethosuximide, 67, 141
Etodolac, 78, 150

Etomidate, 88
Etoposide, 73, 146

Famciclovir, 59, 136
Famotidine, 71, 144
Fazadinium, 88, 158
Felodipine, 33, 110-111
Fenoprofen, 78
Fentanyl, 18, 88, 158
Fexofenadine, 70, 143
Flecainide, 31, 109
Fleroxacin, 53, 130
Fluconazole, 54, 133
Flucytosine, 55, 133
Fludarabine, 74, 146
Flumazenil, 95, 165
Flunarizine, 70, 143
Fluorouracil, 74, 146
Fluoxetine, 96, 167
Flurazepam, 94, 163
Flurbiprofen, 79, 150
Flutamide, 74, 146-147
Fluvastatin, 85, 155
Fluvoxamine, 96, 167
Foscarnet, 59, 136
Fosinopril, 26, 104
Furosemide, 35, 113

Gabapentin, 67, 141
Gallamine, 88, 158
Ganciclovir, 59, 137
Ganciclovir-oral, 59, 137
Gemfibrozil, 85, 155
Gentamicin, 42, 115
Glibornuride, 83
Gliclazide, 83, 154
Glipizide, 83, 154
Glyburide, 83, 154
Glycosides, cardiac, 34, 112
Gold sodium thiomalate, 77, 150
Gout agents, 77-80, 149-152
Griseofulvin, 55, 133
Guanabenz, 24, 102
Guanadrel, 24, 102
Guanethidine, 24
Guanfacine, 25, 103

H_1 antagonists, 69-71, 142-143
H_2 antagonists, 71, 143-144
Haloperidol, 95, 166